Mesothelioma - Diagnostics, Treatment and Basic Research

Edited by Ilze Strumfa

Published in London, United Kingdom

Mesothelioma - Diagnostics, Treatment and Basic Research
http://dx.doi.org/10.5772/intechopen.95137
Edited by Ilze Strumfa

Assistants to the Editor: Romans Uljanovs and Boriss Strumfs

Contributors
Aldo Manuel Alvarez Moran, Jorge Alejandro Torres Ríos, Pablo Alejandro Ávila Sánchez, Lorena Vega Castillo, Venerando Antonio Rapisarda, Caterina Ledda, Nobukazu Fujimoto, Fumie Onishi, Alice Bellini, Beatrice Aramini, Franco Stella, Evdoxia Gogou, Sotirios G. Zarogiannis, Dimitra Siachpazidou, Chryssi Hatzoglou, Konstantinos I. Gourgoulianis, Ave Minajeva, Diana Saranova

First published in London, United Kingdom, 2022 by IntechOpen
IntechOpen is the global imprint of INTECHOPEN LIMITED, registered in England and Wales, registration number: 11086078, 5 Princes Gate Court, London, SW7 2QJ, United Kingdom

British Library Cataloguing-in-Publication Data
A catalogue record for this book is available from the British Library

Additional hard and PDF copies can be obtained from orders@intechopen.com

Mesothelioma - Diagnostics, Treatment and Basic Research
Edited by Ilze Strumfa
p. cm.
Print ISBN 978-1-80355-348-1
Online ISBN 978-1-80355-349-8
eBook (PDF) ISBN 978-1-80355-350-4

Meet the editor

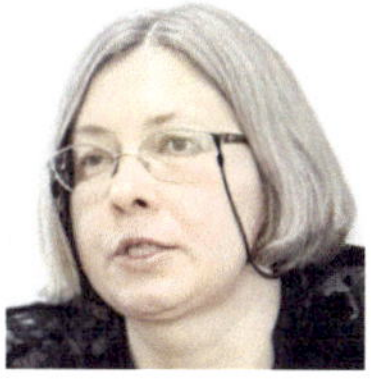

Professor Ilze Strumfa, MD, Ph.D., is an outstanding medical lecturer, actively involved in research in pathology. She graduated from the Medical Academy of Latvia with distinction in 1998, underwent board certification in pathology in 2001, and received a Ph.D. degree in 2005. Currently, she is a professor and head of the Department of Pathology, at Riga Stradins University (RSU), Riga, Latvia. Her 14 years of teaching experience culminated in 2018 in the award of the RSU Lecturer of the Year, given to the most distinguished teachers. As the head of the Department of Pathology, she leads a skilled, motivated team of teachers and scientists whose awards have included Best Academic Unit (2011), Best Ph.D. Student (2012), and Best Digital Junior Teacher (2016). Prof. Strumfa is the author/co-author of more than 100 peer-reviewed journal articles and 16 chapters in scientific monographs/medical textbooks, as well as the editor of three monographs. She has acted as the leading expert in several European and national research projects devoted to the development of diagnostic technologies, laboratory training in research, cancer pathology and tumour microenvironment. Her main research interests include morphological and molecular diagnostics and prognostic assessment of tumours as well as digital pathology and other innovations in pathology and cytology.

Contents

Preface

Mesothelioma is a peculiar malignant tumour that develops from the mesothelial lining of serosal cavities, including pleura (more than 80% of cases), peritoneum, pericardium and tunica vaginalis. It is well known for its classic association with asbestos exposure and unusual gross growth pattern. However, as a difficult diagnosis with limited treatment efficacy and thus adverse survival, mesothelioma also represents an unmet need for the healthcare system. Despite its rarity, mesothelioma remains an intriguing clinical and scientific challenge. As regards basic research, the dominant yet incomplete association with asbestos provides a stable background for pathogenetic studies and search for other causes. Clinically, the possibilities of surgical treatment are limited because of the anatomic fragility of serous membranes and extensive tumour spread; the response to current chemotherapeutic options is unsatisfactory and even the definitive confirmation of diagnosis can be complicated.

Mesothelioma - Diagnostics, Treatment and Basic Research is intended as a summary of classic views and recent advances in pathogenetic concepts, diagnostics, treatment and scientific studies of mesothelioma. It contains a collection of review articles, grouped into three sections: "Etiology and Pathogenesis of Mesothelioma", "Diagnostic Aspects of Mesothelioma" and "Treatment of Mesothelioma".

In the first section, Chapter 1 is devoted to the causes and pathogenesis of malignant mesothelioma, and provides a complete and clear analysis of different etiological agents comprising not only asbestos but also erionite, fluoroedenite, balangeroite and carbon nanotubes, as well as genetic factors, including BAP1 and other genes linked to the pathogenesis of malignant mesothelioma. The authors also discuss the role of simian virus SV 40, ionising radiation and inflammation in the development of mesothelioma. The pathogenesis is further detailed in Chapter 2 on epigenetic events in pleural mesothelioma.

Although the ultimate "gold standard" of mesothelioma diagnostics is verification of the diagnosis in tissue material, this is an invasive approach, hence the search for new technologies. The second section, "Diagnostic Aspects of Mesothelioma", begins with an introduction to the cytological, histological and immuno-phenotypical diagnostics of mesothelioma, covered in Chapter 3. The comprehensive analysis of a complex morphological diagnosis is adapted both for pathologists and clinicians. Recent (2021) changes in WHO classification, as well as morphological features of mesothelioma and relevant immunohistochemical stains, are also discussed. The general mesothelial markers, markers for differential diagnosis between benign versus malignant mesothelial cells, as well as carcinoma markers, are presented. The basic technical requirements and laboratory procedures used for the preparation of cytological and histological samples are also discussed. These aspects are among the major strengths of this chapter because they have been less extensively discussed in previous scientific literature, but can influence the diagnostic outcome significantly.

Chapter 4, by a world-renowned group of scientists who have significantly contributed to current mesothelioma research, looks at diagnostic advances, with an examination of a patient-friendly, innovative approach in the early diagnostics of pleural mesothelioma by assessment of a novel marker, fibulin-3. The gene expression of fibulin-3 is described, followed by an explanation of its biological action and a description of laboratory methods used to detect this molecule in tissues and in biological liquids. Findings in tissue samples, pleural fluid and peripheral blood are reported, and the informativity of fibulin-3 is compared with other biomarkers.

The third section concentrates on surgical and non-surgical treatment of mesothelioma. Surgical approaches to pleural mesothelioma are highlighted in Chapter 5 by a team of experts in this challenging and highly controversial area. The crucial types of operations for mesothelioma – extrapleural pneumonectomy and pleurectomy/decortication – are described and critically analysed, with their indications and outcomes. The role of surgery is discussed within the frameworks of pre-operative diagnostic evaluation and multimodality oncological treatment.

However, mesothelioma is rarely amenable to surgery, leaving systemic therapy as the main treatment approach. Chapter 6 is devoted to developments in systemic cytotoxic treatment, inhibitors of angiogenesis and immune checkpoint inhibitors for the therapy of malignant pleural mesothelioma. Recent mesothelioma trials are summarised in a clear, reader-friendly review. In view of the dismal prognosis of mesothelioma and the limited response to current therapeutic options, the topic is clinically and scientifically important.

The book has been created by a truly global team of doctors and scientists from Italy, Japan, Mexico, Greece and Estonia. We would like to sincerely thank all the authors for their excellent contributions, clinical experience and sharp minds.

This work would not have been possible without the editorial help of my distinguished colleagues, Dr. Romans Uljanovs and Boriss Strumfs, MSc, Ph.D.

Last but not least, we express our sincere gratitude to the IntechOpen editorial team for their continuous support and professional help throughout all stages of book production.

Ilze Strumfa, MD, Ph.D.
Department of Pathology,
Riga Stradiņš University,
Riga, Latvia

Section 1

Etiology and Pathogenesis of Mesothelioma

Chapter 1

Causes and Pathogenesis of Malignant Mesothelioma

Evdoxia Gogou, Sotirios G. Zarogiannis, Dimitra Siachpazidou, Chryssi Hatzoglou and Konstantinos I. Gourgoulianis

Abstract

Malignant mesothelioma (MM) is a malignancy that arises from the mesothelium, a thin layer of tissue that covers the body's serous cavities, such as the pleural, peritoneal, pericardial, and tunica vaginalis of the testis. More than 80% of all mesothelioma cases originate from the pleura and approximately 75–80% of patients are males. It is almost always fatal with most of those affected dying within a year of diagnosis. Asbestos exposure is the most common cause of MM, which mostly affects the pleura. Various factors, including other mineral fibers, carbon nanotubes, or genetic mutations, are also suggested to have a role in the development of MM. The involvement of asbestos, other mineral fibers, nanotechnological products, the simian virus SV40, ionizing radiation, genetic factors, and inflammation in the development of MM has been discussed in this chapter. This study focuses on the role of other mineral fibers, such as erionite, fluoroedenite, balangeroite, and carbon nanotubes, as well as genetic mutations in BAP1 and other genes, in the pathogenesis of MM. The etiology of MM is considered to be complex, and greater knowledge of the pathogenetic pathways may lead to the identification of effective and personalized treatment targets.

Keywords: causes of mesothelioma, pathogenesis of mesothelioma, asbestos, BAP1 mutations, carbon nanotubes, mineral fibers

1. Introduction

Malignant mesothelioma (MM) is a rare and aggressive cancer that affects the mesothelial cells lining the serosal membranes of body cavities, such as the pleura (83% of cases), peritoneum (11%), pericardium, and tunica vaginalis (1–2%) [1–3]. MM is histologically classified into three types—epithelioid accounting for 80% of the cases, sarcomatoid accounting for more than 10%, and biphasic, which has both epithelioid and sarcomatoid features [4, 5]. The epithelioid subtype is associated with a better prognosis compared to sarcomatoid and biphasic subtypes [5, 6]. Histology and TNM (tumor lymph nodes metastasis) staging are the main prognostic factors and the prognosis remains poor with a median survival from 4 to 19 months [5].

A total of 80% of MM cases concern the pleura and the main cause is asbestos exposure [1]. Approximately 50% of patients with MM have a history of prior asbestos exposure [7]. The median age of diagnosis is 75 years of age and the latency period (the period from the initial asbestos exposure until the diagnosis of mesothelioma) is around 30–40 years [8]. The incidence of mesothelioma is still increasing, despite the wide prohibition of asbestos use. Except for asbestos, exposure to other mineral fibers having similar characteristics, such as erionite or fluoro-edenite, has been implicated in the development of MM [1]. A limited number of MMs are attributed to exposure to ionizing radiation for diagnostic or therapeutic purposes. Asbestos has been widely used for decades globally and 10–17% of those highly exposed to asbestos develop MM [9]. This observation has led to the hypothesis that a possible role of genetic risk factors modifies the effect of asbestos exposure [1]. Recent studies have suggested germline mutations in DNA repairs genes, such as BAP1 (BRCA-1-associated protein) in patients with pleural MM [10, 11]. Approximately 21–63% of MMs involve BAP1 somatic or germline mutations, while 22% of patients with BAP1 mutations will develop MM at some point [2].

During the last years, there have been advances in the understanding of the biology and pathogenesis of mesothelioma. The pathogenesis of MM is thought to be multifactorial and a better understanding of the pathogenetic mechanisms may enable the identification of efficient and personalized treatment patterns for precision medicine. The purpose of our study is to present the causes of mesothelioma by enriching them with the latest data and also describe the possible pathogenetic mechanisms for the development of this insidious cancer.

2. Causes of malignant mesothelioma

2.1 Asbestos exposure

The main cause of MM is exposure to air-born asbestos [11, 12]. Asbestos is a silicate mineral classified into two major groups—the amphiboles group that are sharp, needle-like fibers including crocidolite (known as blue asbestos), amosite (brown asbestos), tremolite, actinolite, and anthophyllite, and the serpentines group that are curly fibers, including chrysotile (known as white asbestos) [12–15]. All asbestos fibers are considered as carcinogenic by the WHO and the International Agent for Research on Cancer (IARC) (group 1) [12, 16]. The latency period varies between 20 and 70 years [17, 18].

Asbestos-related mesothelioma cases vary by gender, anatomical region, fiber type, and occupation [19–21]. Most pleural MMs in males are caused by occupational amphibole asbestos exposure. From 2 to 18% of those who were heavily occupationally exposed to amphibole, have developed pleural MM. While the incidence of pleural MM among those occupationally exposed to chrysotile ranges from 0% to 0.47% [19]. Peritoneal MM cases have been reported in those with commercial exposure to amphibole asbestos [22]. However, more recent studies reported that almost 50% of persons with peritoneal MM have fiber load within control values indicating a possible other cause in these tumors [19]. Few studies referred to pericardial or testicular MM and their data did not support the role of asbestos in these sites [23].

The risk of developing MM is related to the type of fiber, the severity, and the duration of exposure [17, 24]. The carcinogenic potency of mineral fibers is determined by the dimensions, durability, dose, and physical properties. Bioavailability after inhalation is affected by fiber dimensions, durability, and dose. Long and thin fibers are associated with higher cytotoxicity and mutagenesis [17, 25]. The WHO distinguished asbestos fibers in short asbestos fibers (SAF) with length < 5 μm and long asbestos fibers (LAF) with length > 5 μm, diameter < 3 μm, and length/diameter ratio > 3 [11, 26]. The longer asbestos fibers, the more carcinogenic potential [26]. Furthermore, fiber biopersistence influences tumorigenesis. The shorter biopersistence, the lower carcinogenic potential as observed in serpentine chrysotile compared with amphiboles and erionite [17]. However, if the exposure to short biopersistence fibers, such as chrysotile, is prolonged, the mesothelial cells could be transformed [27]. MM from occupational asbestos exposure is mainly caused by crocidolite and amosite fibers [28, 29].

The mass mining of asbestos began in the twentieth century and it was mainly used for insulation against heat, fire, and corrosion, while its previous use was in pottery [12]. Thus, high-risk occupations include engineers who work on brake and clutch lining, builders, dockyard and shipyard workers, plumbers, and electricians [4].

Asbestos exposure can occur mainly occupationally for asbestos workers and nonoccupationally including domestic, neighborhood, or environmental exposure [4, 12, 30]. The risk of developing pleural MM after nonoccupational exposure depends on the types of fibers. The risk is greater to amphiboles exposure than to chrysotile [11]. However, it is complicated to establish accurately asbestos exposure. There is unquestionable asbestos exposure in asbestos miners and shipyards workers. Other categories of workers may not correctly remember events that occurred 30–50 years earlier, as the latency period is too long. Specific questionnaires were developed to identify different levels of exposure within occupational asbestos exposure individuals. Another evidence of asbestos exposure is the measurement of lung tissue fiber content, but this is rarely performed as it is invasive, costly, and for legal implications [11, 12]. The combination of a complete occupational history and radiological evidence of exposure, such as bilateral calcified pleural plaques and/or histological evidence of asbestos fibers in lung tissue, could be used to estimate asbestos exposure. For example, pleural plaques were found in 88% of asbestos exposure patients with mesothelioma [11, 29].

Asbestos use was prohibited in most western countries between 1970 and 2005, except for the USA, where it was only partly banned, and Canada, where the asbestos ban was implemented in 2018 [10, 31]. These countries represent 16% of the world's population [12]. Unfortunately, in developing countries, asbestos use and mining are ongoing with an annual worldwide production of about 2.2 million metric tons [32]. Hence, the incidence of MM will continue to increase worldwide [12].

2.1.1 Carcinogenic mechanisms of asbestos

When asbestos and other fibers enter the pleura and peritoneum via lymphatics, they reside there for months or years, triggering a chronic inflammatory response stimulated by high mobility group protein B1 (HMGB1) secretion and related inflammasome activation in mesothelial cells, which activates the nuclear factor kappa-light-chain-enhancer of activated B cells (NF-kB) and phosphatidylinositol 3-kinase (PI3K) [33–36]. This environment promotes the proliferation of mesothelial cells that have spontaneously acquired mutations or are exposed to mutagenic reactive oxygen species generated by inflammatory cells in the area of asbestos deposits [34, 35]. Asbestos-activated macrophages produce reactive oxygen species (ROS), which can cause DNA damage by forming 8-hydroxy-2-deoxyguanosine (8-OHDG) adducts [34]. Ferroptosis, a non-apoptotic, iron-dependent cell death, has recently been linked to asbestos-related carcinogenesis [37]. Hepatocyte growth factor (HGF) may also play a role in asbestos-induced carcinogenesis by activating the PI3K/MEK5/Fra-1 axis (phosphatidylinositol 3-kinase/mitogen/extracellular signal-regulated kinase kinases 5/(Fos-related antigen 1) [38]. Crocidolite and erionite have a longer biopersistence than chrysotile, which explains their greater pathogenicity [35].

Asbestos fibers are phagocytosed by human mesothelial cells, and once inside the cell, they can mechanically interfere with the cell spindle during mitosis, causing chromosomal mutations responsible for carcinogenesis, but this hypothesis has been ruled out [11, 39].

The carcinogenesis mechanism in pleural MM is complex. Inhaled asbestos fibers move to the pleura. Fibers in the pleural space irritate the tissue, resulting in a cycle of tissue injury and repair. When asbestos fibers are phagocytosed by macrophages, oxygen-free radicals are produced, causing intracellular DNA damage and aberrant repair [40]. Asbestos fibers also enter mesothelial cells, interfering with mitosis, causing DNA mutations, and changing chromosome structure. Inflammatory cytokines are released by asbestos-exposed mesothelial cells, including tumor growth factor, platelet-derived growth factor, and vascular endothelial growth factor (VEGF) [40]. This creates an ideal environment for tumor development. Finally, asbestos increases the expression of proto-oncogenes and promotes aberrant cellular proliferation by phosphorylating different protein kinases (mitogen-activated protein and extracellular signal-regulated kinases 1 and 2) [27]. Asbestos fibers are known to cause DNA damage, which is repaired by homologous recombination (HR) and double-strand break repair, mismatch repair system (MMR), and nonhomologous end-joining (NHE) or nucleotide excision repair (NER), putting people with DNA repair faults at a higher risk of developing MM [1, 41–44].

2.2 Erionite

Erionite is a fibrous type of zeolite and according to its physical characteristics, it resembles amphiboles amosite or crocidolite [19, 45]. Chemically, it consists of potassium aluminum silicate with various amounts of calcium and sodium [19]. Deposits of erionite have been described in the Cappadocian region of Turkey, in the intermountain west of the United States from Oregon into Mexico and the Sierra Madre region [46, 47]. High amounts of airborne erionite were found in North Dakota, where miles of roads were surfaced with erionite-containing gravel [48]. Also, erionite has been identified in North-Eastern Italy [49].

Studies have shown that erionite is a carcinogenic fiber that causes the MM epidemic in some Cappadocian villages in Turkey [48, 50]. There, erionite was used to build houses and pave roads. Environmental exposure to erionite fibers was documented not only in Cappadocian of Turkey but also in Mexico, North Dakota, Nevada, and California [46–48, 51]. More specifically, in North Dakota erionite has been used to pave roads, in Nevada referred exposure to asbestos, erionite, and other types of fibers, and in California referred exposure to chrysotile and tremolite [48, 51, 52]. These fibers get released into the air due to human activities, such as mining, road construction, and off-road driving. Environmental exposure often begins at birth and occurs randomly among males and females. That is why MM caused by environmental exposure tends to occur at a younger age < 55 years with a 1:1 male: female, contrary to MM caused by occupational asbestos exposure that has a ratio 3:1 [53]. Mineralogical and pedigree analyses in villages in Cappadocian of Turkey have revealed that in addition to environmental exposure there may also be an autosomal dominant genetic susceptibility to MM [50, 54]. Middle-aged patients diagnosed with mesothelioma in North America reported living in Mexico at a young age and having emigrated. Their fiber burden analysis in lung tissue demonstrated a high aspect ratio of erionite fibers, which existed in high concentrations in Mexico [46, 55]. Experimental animal studies have confirmed the high carcinogenic potential of erionite [56, 57]. Erionite also could cause other disorders, such as mesothelial hyperplasia, dysplasia, and pleural fibrosis [56]. The way erionite is thought to cause MM is by activation of the NLRP3 (NOD-, LRR- and pyrin domain-containing protein 3) inflammasome, which in turn triggers an autocrine feedback loop in mesothelial cells, modulated by the interleukin-1 receptor [58].

2.3 Fluoro-edenite

Fluoro-edenite has similar morphology and composition to actinolite and tremolite. This mineral was extracted from an area located at Southeast of Biancavilla in Catania, Eastern Sicily, Italy. It was used as a building material, for road paving, for residential and commercial plaster, and also for mortar construction [19]. A study showed a 10-fold increase in pleural neoplasms among those exposed to fluoro-edenite [59]. An experimental animal study revealed that when fluoro-edenite was implanted in peritoneal cavities of rats, MM was induced [60]. Fluoro-edenite was classified as Group 1 carcinogenic to humans [61]. According to studies *in vitro*, fluoro-edenite induces DNA damage and leads to the production of reactive oxygen species (ROS) resulting in decreased cell viability [62].

2.4 Balangeroite

Balangeroite is a fibrous iron-rich magnesium silicate and it is often intergrown with chrysotile deposits. Deposits have been found in Balangero in Italy, after which it is named. It has a similar morphology but lower bio-durability than commercial amphiboles [63, 64]. The role of these amphibole mineral fibers in the induction of MM in Balangero in Italy is controversial with some authors attributing MMs to balangeroite and others blurring its precise role [64, 65]. The controversy arises from the fact that some Balangero chrysotile miners have commercial amphiboles (crocidolite and amosite) in the mineral analysis of lung tissue. Also, it was known that the Balangero mines occasionally milled imported commercial amphibole from South Africa [63, 65].

2.5 Other minerals

Other minerals include man-made vitreous fibers, such as rock wool, slag wool, glass fiber and glass filament. All mineral wools are formed by spinning or drawing molten mineral or rock materials, such as slag and ceramics. These are applied to thermal insulation, filtration, soundproofing, and hydroponic medium [66]. The more biopersistent man-made vitreous fibers were classified by IARC (International Agency for Research on Cancer) as "possible carcinogenic to humans" (group 2b) [66]. More biopersistent refractory ceramic fibers have been linked to the induction of MM in Syrian golden hamsters exposed to high-dose chronic inhalation experiments [67]. Some case reports of MM have been related to beryllium, nickel, and crystalline silica, but these data have not been supported by epidemiological studies [19]. There is an increased risk of pleural MM for those exposed to both asbestos and mineral wool or silica according to one study [68].

2.6 Simian Virus 40 (SV40)

SV40 is a DNA polyomavirus that has been reported as a possible etiologic agent for human MM [69]. Human exposure to SV40 occurred between 1955 and 1963 when inactivated and live anti-polio vaccines were administrated to people in the United States, Canada, Europe, Asia, and Africa [70].

SV40 sequences have been found by the polymerase chain reaction (PCR) method in various human cancers, such as MM, non-Hodgkin lymphoma, osteosarcoma, and thyroid tumors [71]. There are data available on the role of SV40 in the pathogenesis of human MM. For example, this virus activates genes promoting cell progression and proliferation, it induces apoptosis of mesothelial cells transfected with antisense DNA to the SV40, and MM harboring SV40 has a poorer prognosis compared to SV40-negative MM [69]. Mesothelial cells are susceptible to infection and transformation by SV40 [72]. The viral genome encodes oncogenic proteins like large T-antigen (Tag), which inactivate the tumor suppressor activity of p53 and p-retinoblastoma family proteins. However, the presence of SV40 DNA and protein in MM has not led to the definitive causal relationship between the virus and MM development [73]. According to some researchers, SV40 in humans may be a passenger virus in the mesothelial cells without causing pathology or tumorigenesis [69]. Overall, the role of SV40 as an etiologic agent in human MM is still in debate.

2.7 Radiation

Ionizing radiation is a high-risk factor for malignancy development. Its effect is cumulative, so once received, the effects remain in the body for life. Individuals with increased levels of exposure to ionizing radiation have a greater risk of malignancies later in their life [74]. The carcinogenic risk associated with exposure to ionizing radiation has been evaluated previously in the IARC monographs [66].

The evidence linking radiation to MM in humans comes—(i) from clinical studies involving patients who had previously received radiotherapy for tumors, (ii) from reported cases of MM occurring after the use of the contrast agent thorotrast, and (iii) from studies of workers exposed to prolonged lower levels of radiation [19]. Cases of pleural, peritoneal, and pericardial mesothelioma have been reported after radiotherapy in childhood or adulthood due to lymphoma, genital, renal, and breast neoplasms [75, 76]. The radiation-induced MMs had a latent period from 5 to 50 years and an equal male: female ratio [77]. The intravenous thorotrast administration has caused not only MM but also hepatocellular carcinoma, hemangioendothelioma, and cholangiocarcinoma. The radioactive Thorotrast ($^{232}ThO_2$) is insoluble and after injection, deposits in organs and is associated with slow decay and prolonged alpha-ray emission [19]. Cases of MM have been reported in radiation technologists and among workers in the atomic energy industry [78]. A genetic analysis study has shown that radiation-induced MMs have copy number gains outnumbering deletions, which are more common in asbestos-induced MMs, signifying potential different molecular mechanisms of induction [79]. Overall, radiation is a risk factor to MM in directly irradiated tissues and to a lesser extent in tissues distant from the target site.

2.8 Chronic inflammation and MM

Chronic serosal membranes inflammations can induce MM of pleura and peritoneum [80]. Therapeutic plombage used as a treatment for pulmonary tuberculosis and longstanding chronic empyema could induce pleural MM. Moreover, recurrent peritonitis as a result of relapsing diverticulitis or Crohn's disease or Familial Mediterranean Fever, ventriculoperitoneal shunts for hydrocephaly have been reported as a cause of peritoneal MM [80, 81]. Chronic interleukin-6 production has been linked to MM pathogenesis as a regulatory cytokine in the acute phase response [19].

2.9 BAP1 (BRCA-1-associated protein 1)

Recently, many researchers are concerned with the role of BAP1 in mesothelioma. BAP1 is a nuclear protein, which is encoded by a tumor suppressor gene (BAP1 gene) located on chromosome 3p21.1 [10, 82]. BAP1 was discovered in 1998 as a novel ubiquitin carboxyl-terminal hydrolase, an enzyme responsible for removing ubiquitin from protein substrates [83]. BAP1 is binding to BRCA1 enhancing its tumor-suppressive activity [7, 83]. Also, BAP1 regulates proteins involved in DNA damage repair, cellular differentiation, chromatin modulation, cell cycle control and cell proliferation, immune regulation, and consequently, it has a tumor-suppressive effect [7]. BAP1 is a nuclear protein that belongs to a family of multiprotein transcriptional regulators that control genes related to metabolism, mitochondrial function, and cell proliferation [33, 37]. The identification of BAP1 as a key regulator of cell death and metabolism aided in the description of the complex set of molecular events mediated by asbestos carcinogenesis [84].

Clinical reports have shown that BAP1 is commonly lost or inactivated in various cancers [85]. An increase in the spontaneous development of breast cancer, lung, ovarian and a few cases of MM that are not related to asbestos in about half of mice with genetically engineered BAP1 mutations that match those found in BAP1 cancer syndrome families supports the idea that BAP1 is a tumor suppressor [86]. BAP1 mutations occur in a wide range of people. According to a study, BAP1 germline mutations were found in 7.7% of spontaneous MM cases [87]. It is suggested that germline mutations in BAP1 are thought to start with just one abnormal allele. Low-level asbestos exposure resulted in second allele mutations in genetically vulnerable hosts, resulting in the development of MM linked to BAP1 [88]. Experiments with animal subjects have backed up the aforementioned theory. Experiments in BAP1+/− mice revealed that after intraperitoneal injection of crocidolite asbestos, animals developed MM at twice the rate of wild-type mice, while no MMs were observed in BAP+/− mice not exposed to asbestos [89]. Other researchers discovered that BAP1 knockout mice developed MM without ever having been exposed to asbestos [86]. Another study presented that none of the patients with MM and gene mutations reported occupational asbestos exposure, highlighting that these tumors were either due to low levels of environmental exposure or not due to exposure to carcinogenic fibers [90]. The same study showed that most patients were female and almost half of the tumors were located in the peritoneum, arguing that they were not related to asbestos exposure, as if the cause was both asbestos exposure and genetic predisposition, then the male: female ratio would be maintained and most tumors would be located in the pleura [90].

Taking into consideration the functional role of BAP1 in many cellular pathways implicated in cancer, it is not surprising that the BAP1 gene is mutated in a variety of tumors [85]. BAP1 mutations observed in cancer are primarily inactivating mutations, such as chromosomal deletions of the BAP1 gene, leading to loss of function. BAP1 mutations occur in both germline and somatic forms [7, 85]. Germline mutations of the BAP1 gene are inherited in an autosomal dominant pattern and constitute a novel tumor predisposition syndrome (BAP1-TPDS) conferring a high risk of hereditary cancers [87, 91]. The cancers associated with this syndrome are MM, uveal or cutaneous melanoma, and renal cell carcinoma [92]. MM is the second most common cancer identified with BAP1-TPDS accounting for 22% of tumors with a median age of onset of 46 years and a seven-fold longer survival rate compared to a patient with sporadic MM [90]. Somatic BAP1 mutations appear in similar types of tumors as in patients with germline mutations. A total of 50% of MM patients were found to have somatic BAP1 mutations and interestingly, they show significantly longer survival than those without mutations on BAP1 [93, 94]. Around 21–63% of MM patients have BAP1 mutations (germline or somatic), and 22% of those who have BAP1 mutations will develop MM. BAP1 genetic mutations are normally present in all cells with one mutant allele, whereas somatic inactivation of a second allele causes cancer [95, 96]. For BAP1 mutation carriers, the gene–environmental interaction is thought to play a key role in cancer susceptibility [95]. In the general population, BAP1 mutations are uncommon, and there are no homozygotes [97]. In distinct cases, their prevalence has been reported to be 1–2% for uveal melanoma, 0.5% for cutaneous melanoma, and 0–7% for MM, rising to 25%, 0.7%, and 20%, respectively, in family cases [43, 44]. In MMs and other malignancies linked to BAP1-TPDS, tumor aggressiveness varies greatly, and the underlying genetic processes are unknown [10].

2.10 Other genes linked to MM pathogenesis

A handful of the genes implicated in chromatin regulation are mutated in MM patients. Some genes [CDKN2A (cyclin-dependent kinase inhibitor 2A gene), TMEM127 (transmembrane protein 127 gene)] encode tumor suppressor proteins involved in cell growth, proliferation, and survival. Other genes, such as NF2 (neurofibromin 2), encode proteins that modulate signaling pathways for modulating cell shape, cell growth, and cell adhesion [10, 98]. Other genes, such as KDR (kinase insert domain receptor), encode vascular endothelial growth factor (VEGF) receptors that increase endothelial cell proliferation, survival, migration, and differentiation [99]. The pathophysiological mechanisms underlying the development of MM as a result of these genetic mutations are still unknown.

Many studies highlight different clinical parameters that can predict the presence of an inherited mutation in MM, such as minimal asbestos exposure, peritoneal disease, young age, and a second cancer diagnosis [42–44]. This finding is significant because it could lead to the development of clinical panel-based genetic testing and the adoption of clinical genetic testing recommendations. For MM patients, genetic testing would be extremely beneficial because it would allow for the early detection and prevention of malignancies in high-risk individuals. The earlier cancers are detected and treated, the better the chances of survival [10].

According to comprehensive Genome-Wide Association Studies (GWAS) on MM, the most significant SNP (single nuclear polymorphisms) were found in genes involved in cell adhesion, migration, and apoptosis, and may promote carcinogenesis via mechanisms triggered by the human immune system's response to asbestos fibers [100]. Reactive oxygen species (ROS) and free radicals, which arise as a result of inhaled asbestos fiber, are thought to have a role in asbestos toxicity and carcinogenicity. Genetic polymorphisms in detoxification genes encode proteins that are involved in the detoxification and clearance of ROS or change enzyme function, which may increase cancer risk. Furthermore, genetic polymorphisms in DNA repair genes result in a deficiency in DNA repair pathways, which fail to defend against the oxidative stress generated by asbestos fibers, ultimately leading to an increased risk of carcinogenesis [101]. Individuals who were homozygotes or heterozygotes in one of four DNA repair genes were more likely to develop pleural MM than controls [10, 99, 101].

Reduced expression of critical molecules in the p53 tumor-suppressor gene pathway, such as p14, p16, and NF2-MERLIN (Moesin-ezrin-radixin-like protein), has been discovered as a result of genetic profiling of pleural MM [27, 102]. Other genes, such as BRCA-associated protein 1 (BAP1), set domain containing 2 (SETD2), unc-like autophagy activating kinase (ULAK2), ryanodine receptor 2 (RR2), cilia and flagella associated protein 45 (CFAP45), and set domain bifurcated 1 (SETDB1), have been shown to have deletions or loss mutations in pleural MM [17].

More research is needed to provide a full picture of the genes that predispose to mesothelioma and their role in the molecular pathways of asbestos carcinogenesis that have been revealed, such as chronic inflammation and altered metabolism.

2.11 The role of genes and environment

Carcinogenesis is frequently linked to somatic gene changes that disrupt DNA repair systems, resulting in an accumulation of DNA damage and an increase in the proportion of cells with damaged DNA. Cancer could arise if these cells kept their survival mechanisms. Inherited mutations affecting DNA repair and other genes may exacerbate carcinogenesis by increasing vulnerability to environmental carcinogens [11, 33]. In the subject of carcinogens, the current method is to explore genes and environment interactions by combining genetic and environmental investigations.

2.12 Carbon nanotubes and mesothelioma

Carbon nanotubes are one-dimensional fibrous nanomaterials that resemble asbestos fibers in their physical properties. In 2014, WHO and IARC (International Agency for Research on Cancer) classified long, rigid multiwall carbon nanotubes as group 2B possibly carcinogenic for humans [61, 103]. Only one type of carbon nanotube was categorized in group 2B-possibly carcinogenic to humans in 2014 and this was a commercial product called "MWCNT-7." (multiwall carbon nanotubes-7) [61, 104, 105]. MWCNT-7 are multiwall carbon nanotubes with a structure comparable to asbestos and are biopersistent [106]. Toxicological investigations in animals showed that some forms of carbon nanotubes can cause MM. In animal experimental models, long, large-diameter, rigid multiwall carbon nanotubes supplied by intraperitoneal or intrascrotal injection or trans-tracheal intrapulmonary spraying were shown to develop MM [106–108]. Longer, rigid multiwall carbon nanotubes translocated to the parietal pleura, causing more inflammation, fibrosis, and localized mesothelial cell proliferation than shorter, thinner agglomerates [89]. Many animal experimental studies have shown similar findings [106, 109]. Asbestos fibers and multiwall carbon nanotubes have physicochemical similarities and differences [103]. The "fiber pathogenicity paradigm" identifies width, length, biopersistence, and mechanical bending stiffness as predictors of pathogenicity and carcinogenicity in carbon nanotubes, or other fibrous nanomaterials, and metallic nanowires [110].

Near the end of the twentieth century, carbon nanotubes were found and manufactured. Composite materials, thin coatings and films, microelectronics, energy storage, environmental remediation, and nanomedicine are all areas where they are used [111]. The Royal Society and Royal Academy of Engineering acknowledged the physical similarities between carbon nanotubes and asbestos fibers in 2004, as well as the potential for human health hazards [112]. Chemical vapor deposition (CVD) is the most common industrial method for producing carbon nanotubes, with transition metals catalyzing the breakdown of a carbon-containing organic vapor. Carbon nanotubes can be discharged as dry powders during the manufacturing and processing phases [110]. The National Institute of Occupational Safety and Health (NIOSH) in the United States has set a recommended exposure limit of 1 $\mu g/m^3$ [113]. To prevent repeating the history of asbestos-related disorders, the ultimate goal is to commercialize nanomaterials while simultaneously considering potential human health risks [103].

2.12.1 Pathogenicity of carbon nanotubes

Some forms of carbon nanotubes resemble asbestos fibers in length and rigidity. Long, thin, biopersistent fibers are thought to enter the pleural space, obstruct clearance through lymphatic stomata on the parietal pleura, and cause frustrated phagocytosis, oxidant generation, and persistent inflammation, ultimately leading to MM [110]. Furthermore, the hydrophobicity of raw carbon nanotubes hampered their dispersion in biological conditions, causing them to clump together in rope-like formations or tangled clumps. These clusters clump together to create discrete multifocal granulomas, which comprise macrophage and fibroblast aggregates [114, 115]. Carbon nanotubes were also found in lymph nodes in the mediastinum. Individual carbon nanotubes may be gradually released from pulmonary agglomerates over time and translocated to the lung interstitium, pleura, and regional lymph nodes. Also, many researchers discovered that inhaling well-aerosolized single or multi-walled carbon nanotubes caused persistent inflammation and fibrosis [106]. Very thin carbon nanotubes are more prone to form tangled agglomerates than thicker, rigid multiwall nanotubes. DNA damage can be caused by short multiwall carbon nanotubes with a length of 1 μm [103, 116].

3. Conclusions

Asbestos exposure is the most common cause of MM, however, genetic factors, such as BAP1 gene mutations and exposure to other minerals fibers or nanotechnology products, have also been linked in recent years. It is possible that genetic and environmental factors interact to cause MM development. Knowing the causes of MM can help with early detection and prevention. Furthermore, studying and comprehending the pathogenetic pathways that contribute to the development of mesothelioma can help to find more targeted and effective treatments, hence prolonging survival.

Acknowledgements

The authors would like to thank Chamou Dimitra for the literature assistance.

Competing interests statement

None.

Author details

Evdoxia Gogou[1,2*], Sotirios G. Zarogiannis[1,2], Dimitra Siachpazidou[2], Chryssi Hatzoglou[1,2] and Konstantinos I. Gourgoulianis[2]

1 Faculty of Medicine, Department of Physiology, University of Thessaly, Larissa, Greece

2 Faculty of Medicine, Department of Respiratory Medicine, University of Thessaly, Larissa, Greece

*Address all correspondence to: egogou@uth.gr

References

[1] Betti M, Aspesi A, Sculco M, Matullo G, Magnani C, Dianzani I. Genetic predisposition for malignant mesothelioma: A concise review. Mutation Research Mutation Research. 2019;**781**:1-10. Available from: https://www.sciencedirect.com/science/article/pii/S1383574218300656

[2] Kato S, Tomson BN, Buys TPH, Elkin SK, Carter JL, Kurzrock R. Genomic landscape of malignant mesotheliomas. Molecular Cancer Therapeutics. 2016;**15**(10):2498-2507

[3] Rusch VW, Giroux D, Kennedy C, Ruffini E, Cangir AK, Rice D, et al. Initial analysis of the international association for the study of lung cancer mesothelioma database. Journal of Thoracic Oncology: Official Publication of the International Association for the Study of Lung Cancer. 2012;**7**(11):1631-1639. DOI: 10.1097/JTO.0b013e31826915f1

[4] Asciak R, George V. Update on biology and management of mesothelioma. European Respiratory Review. 2021;**1**:1-13. DOI: 10.1183/16000617.0226-2020

[5] Brcic L, Kern I. Clinical significance of histologic subtyping of malignant pleural mesothelioma. Translational Lung Cancer Research. 2020;**9**(3):924-933

[6] Galateau-salle F, Churg A, Roggli V, Travis WD, Health W. The 2015 World Health Organization classification of tumors of the pleura: Advances since the 2004 classification. Pleural Malignant Mesothelioma. 2015;**11**(2):142-154

[7] Louie BH, Kurzrock R. BAP1: Not just a BRCA1-associated protein. Cancer Treatment Reviews. 2020;**90**(August):102091. DOI: 10.1016/j.ctrv.2020.102091

[8] Woolhouse I, Bishop L, Darlison L, De Fonseka D, Edey A, Edwards J, et al. British Thoracic Society Guideline for the investigation and management of malignant pleural mesothelioma. Thorax. 2018;**73**:i1-i30

[9] Hodgson JT, Darnton A. The quantitative risks of mesothelioma and lung cancer in relation to asbestos exposure. Annals of Occupational Hygiene. 2000;**44**(8):565-601

[10] Panou V, Røe OD. Inherited genetic mutations and polymorphisms in malignant mesothelioma: A comprehensive review. International Journal of Molecular Sciences. 2020;**21**(12):1-18

[11] Carbone M, Prasad S, PSH A, Richard Alexander HR, Baas P, Fabrizio Bardelli F, et al. Mesothelioma: Scientific clues for prevention, diagnosis, and therapy. CA: A Cancer Journal for Clinicians. 2019;**69**(5):402-429

[12] Røe OD, Stella GM. Malignant pleural mesothelioma: History, controversy and future of a manmade epidemic. European Respiratory Society. 2015;**24**(135):115-131. DOI: 10.1183/09059180.00007014

[13] Stayner L, Welch LS, Lemen R. The worldwide pandemic of asbestos-related diseases. Annual Review of Public Health. 2013;**34**:205-216

[14] Kumagai-Takei N, Lee S, Srinivas B, Shimizu Y, Sada N, Yoshitome K, et al. The effects of asbestos fibers on human T cells. International Journal of Molecular Sciences. 2020;**21**(19):1-13

[15] Sporn TA. Mineralogy of asbestos. In: Tannapfel A, editor. Malignant Mesothelioma Recent Results in Cancer Research. Berlin, Heidelberg: Springer; 189, 2011. DOI: 10.1007/978-3-642-10862-4_1

[16] Arsenic IARC, Metals F. Dusts. IARC Monographs on the Evaluation of Carcinogenic Risks to Humans. 2012;**100**:147-167

[17] Bibby AC, Tsim S, Kanellakis N, Ball H, Talbot DC, Blyth KG, et al. Malignant pleural mesothelioma: An update on investigation, diagnosis and treatment. European Respiratory Society. 2016;**25**(142):472-486. DOI: 10.1183/16000617.0063-2016

[18] Robinson BM. Malignant pleural mesothelioma: An epidemiological perspective. The Annals of Cardiothoracic Surgery. 2012;**1**(4):491-496

[19] Attanoos RL, Churg A, Galateau-Salle F, Gibbs AR, Roggli VL. Malignant mesothelioma and its non-asbestos causes. Archives of Pathology & Laboratory Medicine. 2018;**142**(6):753-760

[20] Spirtas R, Heineman EF, Bernstein L, Beebe GW, Keehn RJ, Stark A, et al. Malignant mesothelioma: Attributable risk of asbestos exposure. Occupational and Environmental Medicine. 1994;**51**(12):804-811

[21] Rake C, Gilham C, Hatch J, Darnton A, Hodgson J, Peto J. Occupational, domestic and environmental mesothelioma risks in the British population: A case-control study. British Journal of Cancer. 2009;**100**(7):1175-1183

[22] Browne K, Smither WJ. Asbestos-related mesothelioma: Factors discriminating between pleural and peritoneal sites. British Journal of Industrial Medicine. 1983;**40**(2):145-152

[23] Lowry SJ, Weiss NS. Geographic distribution of incidence of pericardial and paratesticular mesotheliomas in the USA. Cancer Causes Control. 2016;**27**:1487-1489. DOI: 10.1007/s10552-016-0825-3

[24] Wiggins J, Brilton MG, Darlison L, Entwisle J, Greenstone MA, Hetzel M, et al. BTS statement on malignant mesothelioma in the UK, 2007. Thorax. 2007;**62**(Suppl. 2):1-19

[25] Beckett P, Edwards J, Fennell D, Hubbard R, Woolhouse I, Peake MD. Demographics, management and survival of patients with malignant pleural mesothelioma in the National Lung Cancer Audit in England and Wales. Lung Cancer. 2015;**88**(3):344-348. DOI: 10.1016/j.lungcan.2015.03.005

[26] Pierce JS, McKinley MA, Paustenbach DJ, Finley BL. An evaluation of reported no-effect chrysotile asbestos exposures for lung cancer and mesothelioma. Critical Reviews in Toxicology. 2008;**38**(3):191-214

[27] Robinson BWS, Lake RA. Advances in malignant mesothelioma. The New England Journal of Medicine. 2005;**353**(15):1591-1603

[28] Sluis-Cremer GK, Liddell FDK, Logan WPD, Bezuidenhout BN. The mortality of amphibole miners in South Africa, 1946-80. British Journal of Industrial Medicine. 1992;**49**(8):566-575

[29] Dodson RF, O'Sullivan M, Corn CJ, McLarty JW, Hammar SP. Analysis of asbestos fiber burden in lung tissue from mesothelioma patients. Ultrastructural Pathology. 1997;**21**(4):321-336

[30] Panou V, Vyberg M, Meristoudis C, Hansen J, Bøgsted M, Omland Ø, et al.

Non-occupational exposure to asbestos is the main cause of malignant mesothelioma in women in North Jutland, Denmark. Scandinavian Journal of Work, Environment & Health. 2019;**45**(1):82-89

[31] Ruff K. How Canada changed from exporting asbestos to banning asbestos: The challenges that had to be overcome. International Journal of Environmental Research and Public Health. 2017;**14**(10):1135

[32] Hashim D, Boffetta P. Occupational and environmental exposures and cancers in developing countries. Annals of Global Health. 2014;**80**(5):393-411. DOI: 10.1016/j.aogh.2014.10.002

[33] Gaudino G, Xue J, Yang H. How asbestos and other fibers cause mesothelioma. Translational Lung Cancer Research. 2020;**9**(I):S39-S46

[34] Xu A, Wu LJ, Santella RM, Hei TK. Role of oxyradicals in mutagenicity and DNA damage induced by crocidolite asbestos in mammalian cells. Cancer Research. 1999;**59**(23):5922-5926

[35] Qi F, Okimoto G, Jube S, Napolitano A, Pass HI, Laczko R, et al. Continuous exposure to chrysotile asbestos can cause transformation of human mesothelial cells via HMGB1 and TNF-α signaling. The American Journal of Pathology. 2013;**183**(5):1654-1666. DOI: 10.1016/j.ajpath.2013.07.029

[36] Carbone M, Yang H. Targeting mechanisms of asbestos and erionite carcinogenesis in mesothelioma. Clinical Cancer Research. 2012;**18**(3):598-604

[37] Toyokuni S. Iron addiction with ferroptosis-resistance in asbestos-induced mesothelial carcinogenesis: Toward the era of mesothelioma prevention. Free Radical Biology and Medicine. 2019;**133**:206-215. DOI: 10.1016/j.freeradbiomed.2018.10.401

[38] Ramos-Nino ME, Blumen SR, Sabo-Attwood T, Pass H, Carbone M, Testa JR, et al. HGF mediates cell proliferation of human mesothelioma cells through a PI3K/MEK5/Fra-1 pathway. American Journal of Respiratory Cell and Molecular Biology. 2008;**38**(2):209-217

[39] Olofsson KMJ. Specificity of asbestos-induced chromosomal aberrations in short-term cultured human mesothelial cells. Cancer Genetics and Cytogenetics. 1989;**41**(1):33-39. DOI: 10.1016/0165-4608(89)90105-2

[40] Sekido Y. Molecular pathogenesis of malignant mesothelioma. Carcinogenesis. 2013;**34**(7):1413-1419

[41] Toumpanakis DTSE. DNA repair systems in malignant mesothelioma. Cancer Letter. 2011;**312**(2):143-149. DOI: 10.1016/j.canlet.2011.08.021

[42] Pastorino S, Yoshikawa Y, Pass HI, Emi M, Nasu M, Pagano I, et al. A subset of mesotheliomas with improved survival occurring in carriers of BAP1 and other germline mutations. Journal of Clinical Oncology. 2018;**36**(35):3485-3494

[43] Panou V, Gadiraju M, Wolin A, Weipert CM, Skarda E, Husain AN, et al. Frequency of germline mutations in cancer susceptibility genes in malignant mesothelioma. Journal of Clinical Oncology. 2018;**36**(28):2863-2871

[44] Hassan R, Morrow B, Thomas A, Walsh T, Lee MK, Gulsuner S, et al. Inherited predisposition to malignant mesothelioma and overall survival following platinum chemotherapy.

Proceedings of the National Academy of Sciences of the United States of America. 2019;**116**(18):9008-9013

[45] Dogan AU, Dogan M, Hoskins JA. Erionite series minerals: Mineralogical and carcinogenic properties. Environmental Geochemistry and Health. 2008;**30**(4):367-381

[46] Ortega-Guerrero MA, Carrasco-Núñez G. Environmental occurrence, origin, physical and geochemical properties, and carcinogenic potential of erionite near San Miguel de Allende, Mexico. Environmental Geochemistry and Health. 2014;**36**(3):517-529

[47] Baris YI, Grandjean P. Prospective study of mesothelioma mortality in Turkish villages with exposure to fibrous zeolite. Journal of the National Cancer Institute. 2006;**98**(6):414-417

[48] Carbone M, Baris YI, Bertino P, Brass B, Comertpay S, Dogan AU, et al. Erionite exposure in North Dakota and Turkish villages with mesothelioma. Proceedings of the National Academy of Sciences of the United States of America. 2011;**108**(33):13618-13623

[49] Giordani M, Mattioli M, Ballirano P, Pacella A, Cenni M, Boscardin MVL. Geological occurrence, mineralogical characterization, and risk assessment of potentially carcinogenic erionite in Italy. Journal of Toxicology and Environmental Health, Part B. 2017;**20**(2):81-103

[50] Metintas M, Hillerdal G, Metintas S. Malignant mesothelioma due to environmental exposure to erionite: Follow-up of a Turkish emigrant cohort. The European Respiratory Journal. 1999;**13**(3):523-526

[51] Pan XL, Day HW, Wang W, Beckett LA, Schenker MB. Residential proximity to naturally occurring asbestos and mesothelioma risk in California. American Journal of Respiratory and Critical Care Medicine. 2005;**172**(8):1019-1025

[52] Baumann F, Buck BJ, Metcalf RV, Mclaurin BT, Merkler DJ, Carbone M. The presence of asbestos in the natural environment is likely related to mesothelioma in young individuals and women from southern Nevada. Journal of Thoracic Oncology. 2015;**10**(5):731-737

[53] Baumann FCM. Environmental risk of mesothelioma in the United States: An emerging concern-epidemiological issues. Journal of Toxicology and Environmental Health, Part B. 2016;**19**(5-6):231-249

[54] Roushdy-Hammady I, Siegel J, Emri S, Testa JR, Carbone M. Genetic-susceptibility factor and malignant mesothelioma in the Cappadocian region of Turkey. Lancet. 2001;**357**(9254):444-445

[55] Oczypok EA, Sanchez MS, Van Orden DR, Berry GJ, Pourtabib K, Gunter ME, et al. Erionite-associated malignant pleural mesothelioma in Mexico. International Journal of Clinical and Experimental Pathology. 2016;**9**(5):5722-5732

[56] Fraire AE, Lach-Pasko E, Greenberg D, Spjut HJ, Dodson RF, Williams G. Effect of erionite on the pleural mesothelium of the fischer 344 Rat. Laboratory Animal Investigation. 1997;**111**(5):1375-1380. DOI: 10.1378/chest.111.5.1375

[57] Ozesmi M, Patiroglu TE, Hillerdal G, Ozesmi C. Peritoneal mesothelioma and malignant lymphoma in mice caused by fibrous zeolite. British Journal of Industrial Medicine. 1985;**42**(11):746-749

[58] Hillegass JM, Miller JM, MacPherson MB, Westbom CM, Sayan M, Thompson JK, et al. Asbestos and erionite prime and activate the NLRP3 inflammasome that stimulates autocrine cytokine release in human mesothelial cells. Particle and Fibre Toxicology. 2013;**10**(1):1-14

[59] Paoletti I, Batisti D, Bruno C, Di Paola M, Gianfagna AM, Mastrantonio M, et al. Unusually high incidence of malignant pleural mesothelioma in a town of eastern Sicily: An epidemiological and environmental study. Archives of Environmental Health. 2000;**55**(6):392-398

[60] Suzuki YKN. Malignant mesothelioma induced by asbestos and zeolite in the mouse peritoneal cavity. Environmental Research. 1984;**35**(1):277-292. DOI: 10.1016/0013-9351(84)90136-1

[61] Grosse Y, Loomis D, Guyton KZ, Lauby-Secretan B, El Ghissassi F, Bouvard V, et al. International Agency for Research on Cancer Monograph Working Group. Carcinogenicity of fluoro-edenite, silicon carbide fibres and whiskers, and carbon nanotubes. The Lancet Oncology. 2014;**15**(13):1427-1428

[62] Cardile V, Renis M, Scifo C, Lombardo L, Gulino R, Mancari B. PA. Behaviour of the new asbestos amphibole fluoro-edenite in different lung cell systems. The International Journal of Biochemistry & Cell Biology. 2004;**36**(5):849-860. DOI: 10.1016/j.biocel.2003.09.007

[63] Turci F, Tomatis M, Gazzano E, Riganti C, Martra G, Bosia A, et al. FB. Potential toxicity of nonregulated asbestiform minerals: Balangeroite from the western Alps. Part 2: Oxidant activity of the fibers. Journal of Toxicology and Environmental Health, Part A. 2005;**68**(1):21-39

[64] Turci F, Tomatis M, Compagnoni R, Fubini B. Role of associated mineral fibres in chrysotile asbestos health effects: The case of balangeroite. The Annals of Occupational Hygiene. 2009;**53**(5):491-497

[65] Piolatto G, Negri E, La Vecchia C, Pira E, Decarli A, Peto J. An update of cancer mortality among chrysotile asbestos miners in Balangero, northern Italy. British Journal of Industrial Medicine. 1990;**47**(12):810-814

[66] IARC Working Group on the Evaluation of Carcinogenic Risks to. IARC Monographs on the Evaluation of Carcinogenic Risks to Humans. Lyon: IARC; 1988. pp. 39-153

[67] Mast RW, Hesterberg TW, Glass LR, McConnell EE, Anderson R, Bernstein DM. Chronic inhalation and biopersistence of refractory ceramic fiber in rats and hamsters. Environmental Health Perspectives. 1994;**102**(Suppl. 5): 207-209

[68] Lacourt A, Gramond C, Audignon S, Ducamp S, Févotte J, Ilg AGS, et al. Pleural mesothelioma and occupational coexposure to asbestos, mineral wool, and silica. American Journal of Respiratory and Critical Care Medicine. 2013;**187**(9):977-982

[69] Martini F, Corallini A, Balatti V, Sabbioni S, PC& TM. Simian virus 40 in humans. Infect Agents Cancer. 2007;**2**:13-25. DOI: 10.1186/1750-9378-2-13

[70] Shah KNN. Human exposure to SV40: Review and comment. American Journal of Epidemiology. 1976;**103**(1):12

[71] Rotondo JC, Mazzoni E, Bononi I, Tognon M, Martini F. Association between simian virus 40 and human tumors. Frontiers in Oncology. 2019;**9**(July):1-19

[72] Cacciotti P, Libener R, Betta P, Martini F, Porta C, Procopio A, et al. SV40 replication in human mesothelial cells induces HGF/Met receptor activation: A model for viral-related carcinogenesis of human malignant mesothelioma. Proceedings of the National Academy of Sciences of the United States of America. 2001;**98**(21):12032-12037

[73] Manfredi JJ, Dong J, Liu WJ, Resnick-Silverman L, Qiao R, Chahinian P, et al. Evidence against a role for SV40 in human mesothelioma. Cancer Research. 2005;**65**(7):2602-2609

[74] Giuranno L, Ient J, De Ruysscher D, Vooijs MA. Radiation-induced lung injury (RILI). Frontiers in Oncology. 2019;**9**:1-16

[75] Small GR, Nicolson M, Buchan K, Broadhurst P. Pericardial malignant mesothelioma: A latent complication of radiotherapy? European Journal of Cardio-Thoracic Surgery. 2008;**33**(4):745-747

[76] Li X, Brownlee NA, Sporn TA, Mahar A, Roggli VL. Malignant (diffuse) mesothelioma in patients with hematologic malignancies: A clinicopathologic study of 45 cases. Archives of Pathology & Laboratory Medicine. 2015;**139**(9):1129-1136

[77] Roggli VL, Oury TD. MEJ. Malignant mesothelioma in women. Anatomic Pathology. 1997;**2**:147-163

[78] Horie A, Hiraoka K, Yamamoto O, Haratake J, Tsuchiya T. SH. An autopsy case of peritoneal malignant mesothelioma in a radiation technologist. Acta Pathologica Japonica. 1990;**40**(1):57-62

[79] Borczuk AC, Pei J, Taub RN, Levy B, Nahum O, Chen J, et al. Genome-wide analysis of abdominal and pleural malignant mesothelioma with DNA arrays reveals both common and distinct regions of copy number alteration. Cancer Biology Therapy. 2016;**17**(3):328-335. DOI: 10.1080/15384047.2016.1145850

[80] Kodama Y, Hoshi S, Minami M, Kiso M, Takezawa T, Arai T, et al. Malignant mesothelioma associated with chronic empyema with elevation of serum CYFRA19: A case report. Bioscience Trends. 2008;**2**(6):250-254

[81] Livneh A, Langevitz P. PM. Pulmonary associations in familial Mediterranean fever. Current Opinion in Pulmonary Medicine. 1999;**5**(5):326-331

[82] Carbone M, Yang H, Pass HI, Krausz T, Testa JR, Gaudino G. BAP1 and cancer chromosome microarray and genetic linkage analyses on the L and W families implicated. Nature Reviews Cancer. 2014;**13**(3):153-159

[83] Jensen DE, Proctor M, Marquis ST, Gardner HP, Ha SI, Chodosh LA, et al. BAP1: A novel ubiquitin hydrolase which binds to the BRCA1 RING finger and enhances BRCA1-mediated cell growth suppression. Oncogene. 1998;**16**(9):1097-1112

[84] Bononi A, Giorgi C, Patergnani S, Larson D, Verbruggen K, Tanji M, et al. BAP1 regulates IP3R3-mediated Ca2+ flux to mitochondria suppressing cell transformation. Nature. 2017;**546**(7659):549-553

[85] Murali R, Wiesner T, Scolyer RA. Tumours associated with BAP1 mutations. Pathology. 2013;**45**(2): 116-126

[86] Kadariya Y, Cheung M, Xu J, Pei J, Sementino E, Menges CW, et al. Bap1 is a bona fide tumor suppressor: Genetic evidence from mouse models carrying

heterozygous germline Bap1 mutations. Cancer Research. 2016;**76**(9):2836-2844

[87] Testa JR, Cheung M, Pei J, Below JE, Tan Y, Sementino E, et al. Germline BAP1 mutations predispose to malignant mesothelioma. Nature Genetics. 2012;**43**(10):1022-1025

[88] Ohar JA, Cheung M, Talarchek J, Howard SE, Howard TD, Hesdorffer M, et al. Germline BAP1 mutational landscape of asbestos-exposed malignant mesothelioma patients with family history of cancer. Cancer Research. 2016;**76**(2):206-215

[89] Xu J, Kadariya Y, Cheung M, Pei J, Talarchek J, Peng H, et al. Germline mutation of Bap1 accelerates development of Asbestos-induced malignant mesothelioma. Cancer Research. 2014;**74**(16):4388-4397

[90] Baumann F, Flores E, Napolitano A, Kanodia S, Taioli E, Pass H, et al. Mesothelioma patients with germline BAP1 mutations have 7-fold improved long-term survival. Carcinogenesis. 2015;**36**(1):76-81

[91] Wiesner T, Obenauf AC, Murali R, Fried I, Griewank KG, Ulz P, et al. Germline mutations in BAP1 predispose to melanocytic tumors. Nature Genetics. 2011;**43**(10):1018-1022

[92] Tsao H. Genotypic and phenotypic features of BAP1 cancer syndrome: A report of 8 new families and review of cases in the literature. JAMA Dermatology. 2017;**153**(10):999-1006

[93] Farzin M, Toon CW, Clarkson A, Sioson L, Watson N, Andrici J, et al. Loss of expression of BAP1 predicts longer survival in mesothelioma. Pathology. 2015;**47**(4):302-307

[94] Nasu M, Emi M, Pastorino S, Tanji M, Powers A, Luk H, et al. High incidence of somatic BAP1 alterations in sporadic malignant mesothelioma masaki. Journal of Thoracic Oncology. 2015;**10**(4):565-576

[95] Klebe S, Driml J, Nasu M, Pastorino S, Zangiabadi A, Henderson D, et al. BAP1 hereditary cancer predisposition syndrome: A case report and review of literature. Biomarker Research. 2015;**3**(1):1-7

[96] Rai K, Pilarski R, Cebulla CM, Cancer C, Science V, State TO, et al. Comprehensive review of BAP1 tumor predisposition syndrome. Clinical Genetics. 2016;**89**(3):285-294

[97] Karczewski KJ, Francioli LC, Tiao G, Cummings BB, Alföldi J, Wang Q, et al. The mutational constraint spectrum quantified from variation in 141,456 humans. Nature. 2020;**581**(7809): 434-443

[98] Zhang N, Bai H, David KK, Dong J, Zheng Y, Cai J, et al. The Merlin/NF2 tumor suppressor functions through the YAP oncoprotein to regulate tissue homeostasis in mammals. Developmental Cell. 2010;**19**(1):27-38

[99] Kanno S, Oda N, Abe M, Terai Y, Ito M, Shitara K, et al. Roles of two VEGF receptors, Flt-1 and KDR, in the signal transduction of VEGF effects in human vascular endothelial cells. Oncogene. 2000;**19**(17):2138-2146

[100] Matullo G, Guarrera S, Betti M, Fiorito G, Ferrante D, Voglino F, et al. Genetic variants associated with increased risk of malignant pleural mesothelioma: A genome-wide association study. PLoS One. 2013;**8**(4):e61253

[101] Cugliari G, Catalano C, Guarrera S, Allione A, Casalone E, Russo A, et al. DNA methylation of FKBP5 as predictor

of overall survival in malignant pleural mesothelioma. Cancers (Basel). 2020;**12**(11):1-14

[102] Petrilli AM, Fernández-Valle C. Role of Merlin/NF2 inactivation in tumor biology. Oncogene. 2016;**35**(5):537-548

[103] Kane AB, Hurt RH, Gao H. The Asbestos-carbon nanotube analogy: An update. Toxicology and Applied Pharmacology. 2018;**361**:68-80

[104] IARC. IARC Working Group on the Evaluation of Carcinogenic Risks to Humans. IARC Monographs on the Evaluation of Carcinogenic Risks to Humans. Ingested Nitrate and Nitrite, and Cyanobacterial Peptide Toxins. Vol. 94, IARC Monographs on the Evaluation of Carcinogenic Risks to Humans. Lyon: World Health Organization, International Agency for Research on Cancer; 2010

[105] IARC. IARC Monographs on the Evaluation of Carcinogenic. Some Nanomaterials and Some Fibres. Vol. 111, IARC Monographs on the Evaluation of Carcinogenic Risks to Humans. Lyon: World Health Organization, International Agency for Research on Cancer; 2017

[106] Numano T, Higuchi H, Alexander DB, Alexander WT, Abdelgied M, El-Gazzar AM, et al. MWCNT-7 administered to the lung by intratracheal instillation induces development of pleural mesothelioma in F344 rats. Cancer Science. 2019;**110**(8):2485-2492

[107] Sakamoto Y, Nakae D, Fukumori N, Tayama K, Maekawa A, Imai K, et al. Induction of mesothelioma by a single intrascrotal administration of multi-wall carbon nanotube in intact male Fischer 344 rats. The Journal of Toxicological Sciences. 2009;**34**(1):65-76

[108] Takagi A, Hirose A, Nishimura T, Fukumori N, Ogata A, Ohashi N, et al. Induction of mesothelioma in p53+/− mouse by intraperitoneal application of multi-wall carbon nanotube. The Journal of Toxicological Sciences. 2008;**33**(1):105-116

[109] Muller J, Delos M, Panin N, Rabolli V, Huaux F, Lison D. Absence of carcinogenic response to multiwall carbon nanotubes in a 2-year bioassay in the peritoneal cavity of the rat. Toxicological Sciences. 2009;**110**(2):442-448

[110] Donaldson K, Murphy FA, Duffin R, Poland CA. Asbestos, carbon nanotubes and the pleural mesothelium: A review of the hypothesis regarding the role of long fibre retention in the parietal pleura, inflammation and mesothelioma. Particle and Fibre Toxicology. 2010;**7**:1-17

[111] Vance ME, Kuiken T, Vejerano EP, McGinnis SP, Hochella MF, Hull DR. Nanotechnology in the real world: Redeveloping the nanomaterial consumer products inventory. Beilstein Journal of Nanotechnology. 2015;**6**(1):1769-1780

[112] Dowling A, Clift R, Grobert N, Hutton D, Oliver R, O'neill O, et al. Nanoscience and nanotechnologies: Opportunities and uncertainties. London The Royal Society & The Royal Academy of Engineering. 2004;**46**(July):618-618

[113] Dahm MM, Schubauer-Berigan MK, Evans DE, Birch ME, Fernback JE, Deddens JA. Carbon nanotube and nanofiber exposure assessments: An analysis of 14 site visits. The Annals of Occupational Hygiene. 2015;**59**(6):705-723

[114] Ma-Hock L, Strauss V, Treumann S, Küttler K, Wohlleben W, Hofmann T, et al. Comparative inhalation toxicity of multi-wall carbon nanotubes,

graphene, graphite nanoplatelets and low surface carbon black. Particle and Fibre Toxicology. 2013;**10**(1):1-20

[115] Jagirdar RM, Papazoglou ED, Pitaraki E, Kouliou OA, Rouka E, Giannakou L, et al. Cell and extracellular matrix interaction models in benign-mesothelial and malignant pleural mesothelioma cells in 2D and 3D in-vitro. Clinical and Experimental Pharmacology & Physiology. 2021;**48**(4):543-552

[116] Kuempel ED, Jaurand M, Morimoto Y, Pinkerton KE, Sargent LM, Vermeulen RCH, et al. Evaluating the mechanistic evidence and key data gaps in assessing the potential carcinogenicity of carbon nanotubes and nanofibers in humans. Critical Reviews in Toxicology. 2017;**47**(1):1-58

Chapter 2

Epigenomics in Malignant Pleural Mesothelioma

Aldo Manuel Alvarez Moran, Pablo Alejandro Ávila Sánchez, Jorge Alejandro Torres Ríos and Lorena Vega Castillo

Abstract

Malignant pleural mesothelioma (MPM) is a tumor with a relatively low incidence, but whose carcinogenesis, for the most part, involves epigenetic factors that keep its heterogeneity and sometimes are a therapeutic target or an obstacle to the effectiveness of the newest treatments. This chapter summarizes the principal epigenetic dysregulation mechanisms involved in the MPM pathogenesis. The most studied mechanism is hypermethylation mediated by DNA methyltransferases (DNMTs) in different tumor suppressor genes, and the relation with asbestos fiber exposure, which represents the main risk factor. Physiopathology is related to chronic inflammation mediated by free radicals that produce chromosomal alterations, genomic instability, increased angiogenesis, and tumor invasion factors like EGFR, FGFR, TGF-B, and PDGF. Additionally, independent methylation pathways that produce gene silencing such as polycomb complex and SWI/SNF mutation are reviewed. Finally, other mechanisms are described such as hypomethylation with imprint loss and pro-oncogenic gene activation that induce immunological responses, as well as acetylation, deacetylation, and demethylation in the chromatin and histone context.

Keywords: malignant pleural mesothelioma, epigenetics, hypermethylation, asbestos, genomic instability

1. Introduction

Human malignant pleural mesothelioma (MPM) is an invariably fatal tumor due to its heterogeneity, growing from the serous surfaces of the pleura. Many factors are involved in its occurrence, such as exposure to asbestos fibers and simian virus 40; these factors being those that are strongly associated with the tumorigenesis of this disease. The annual incidence of MPM is relatively low, estimated in a range of 0.6–30/10,00,000, but the global occurrence is expected to increase continuously in future years [1]. MPM is extremely heterogeneous in its morphology and molecular phenotypes. The latency period for MPM development is 10–50 years after asbestos exposure. The prognosis for MPM is generally poor, with a median survival time of 12 months from diagnosis [1].

Intratumor heterogeneity refers to a mixture of phenotypic, functional, and genetic differences within cancer cells with various differentiation or hierarchical statuses within the tumor. It is a common feature in most tumors. This heterogeneity has been considered the greatest obstacle to the effectiveness of most cancer therapies, manifesting itself in its sensitivity to different therapies. Several studies have been focused on genetic alterations as part of the mechanism of tumoral cells for the generation and maintenance of this heterogeneity. In addition, some other studies show the role of epigenetic modifications involved in its heterogeneity. Despite this, there is scarce information about epigenetic modifications that could explain this process [1, 2].

Epigenetic modifications are heritable and stable alterations of genes that do not change the DNA sequence, including DNA methylation, histone modification, and non-coding RNA interference modifications. DNA methylation has been extensively studied in the development of cancer. On the one hand, hypermethylation in cancer-related promoter genes induces the silencing or downregulation of tumor suppressor genes and repair genes. On the other hand, hypomethylation of DNA leads to activation of oncogenes and genomic instability. Several authors suggest that aberration in DNA methylation may play an important role on tumor cells heterogeneity [3–5].

The exact mechanisms by which asbestos fibers promote the development of cancer are unknown, however, the most accepted theory is the induction of chronic inflammation and signaling pathways in the transformation of reactive oxygen species generated by asbestos fibers. Therefore, this chapter will address an overview of the epigenetic profile of MPM and the mechanisms that promote epigenetic modifications where asbestos fibers might play an important role.

2. Asbestos-induced molecular alterations

As previously mentioned, asbestos exposure is a primary cause of the development of pleural mesothelioma. Molecular analyses show that asbestos-related carcinogenesis is caused by chronic inflammation that both promote the release of oxygen free radicals that alter intracellular components, and DNA mutation and its consequent transformation. Asbestos fibers also contain iron ions and can induce hemolysis by sequestering iron from hemoglobin. This is particularly important since free iron disproportionately releases H_2O_2, which consequently releases hydroxyl radicals (OH) that oxidize DNA, and release nucleic acids, proteins, and lipids. This process is exacerbated by the release of cytokines including tumor necrosis factor-alpha from macrophages and high mobility of box group 1 (HMGB1) proteins from necrotic cells, leading to an amplification of the inflammatory response and an increase in cells that are driven to oxidative damage. Damaged oxidized DNA, if not properly repaired, is highly mutagenic and can lead to genomic instability. A multitude of oxidative DNA lesions includes oxidation of DNA bases, baseless sites, single-strand breaking, double-strand breaking, and interchain breaking, all of which require different pathways for proper repair. These last two chain-breaking types are particularly toxic, since they cause replication collapse, as well as allow chromosome rearrangements, chromosome gains, losses, or fragmentation [2].

There are other mechanisms involved in how asbestos fibers cause MPM (**Figure 1**). Four proposed models related to asbestos fibers induce genetic and cellular damage to cells, in addition to the previously mentioned chronic inflammation. The different molecular models involved in asbestos exposure are explained below:

I. Reactive oxygen species generated by asbestos fibers with their surface exposed leads to DNA damage and cell membrane rupture. Macrophages that

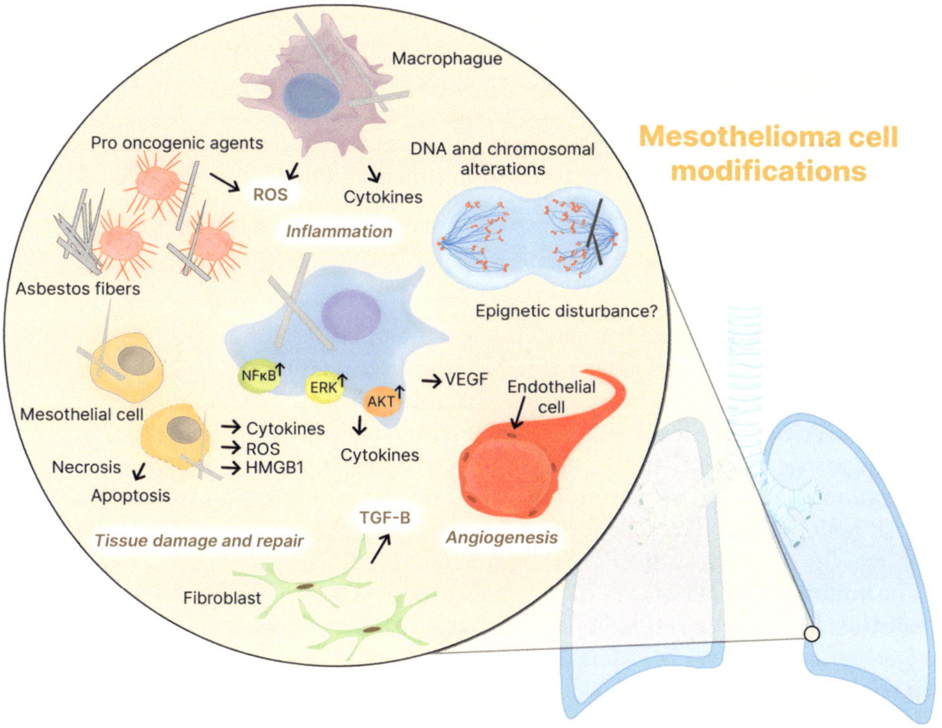

Figure 1.
Possible oncogenic mechanisms induced by asbestos. Abbreviations: HMGB1 = high-mobility group box 1. ROS = reactive oxygen species. TGF-B = transforming growth factor beta. VEGF = vascular endothelial growth factor.

engulf asbestos fibers but cannot digest them also produce abundant reactive oxygen species.

II. Asbestos fibers are also engulfed by mesothelial cells. Asbestos fibers collected in cells can physically interfere with the mitotic process of the cell. The cycle is cut by the interruption of the mitotic spindles. Another important aspect is the entanglement of asbestos fibers with the chromosomes or mitotic spindles that can give rise to structurally damaged chromosomes such as aneuploidies of normal mesothelial cells.

III. Asbestos fibers can absorb a variety of proteins and chemicals on the wide surface of asbestos, which can result in the accumulation of dangerous molecules including carcinogens. The asbestos fibers also bind to important cellular proteins and a deficiency of these proteins can also be detrimental to normal mesothelial cells.

IV. Finally, mesothelial cells and macrophages exposed to asbestos release a variety of cytokines and growth factors that induce inflammation and tumor promotion. These include tumor necrosis factor α, interleukin 1β, transforming growth factor β, and platelet-derived growth factor. Tumor necrosis factor-α has been shown to activate nuclear factor-κB, leading to mesothelial cell survival and inhibiting asbestos-induced cytotoxicity. The high mobility group protein box 1

(GAMB1) is released from mesothelial cells, which are exposed to asbestos and then undergo necrotic cell death, promoting an inflammatory response. Thus, aberrantly activated signaling between mesothelial cells, inflammatory cells, fibroblasts, and other stromal cells can create a set of mesothelial cells, which harbor aneuploidy and DNA damage, potentially developing cancer cells and together all these phenomena form a tumoral microenvironment that supports and nurtures them [6–8].

2.1 DNA methylation

Methylated DNA studied through immunoprecipitation grounded on next-generation sequencing makes it possible to analyze the DNA methylome, which constitutes a useful and efficient tool in the approach of cancer epigenomics [5, 9, 10].

An important and widely described phenomenon in the development of MPM is the epigenetic dysregulation that promotes changes in gene expression [11]. DNA methylation modifications play an important role in the malignant transformation of mesothelioma. Survival in MPM has been attributed to promoter methylation and silencing of genes such as SFRP4, SFRP5, FHIT, and SLCA20.

The methylated CpG islands have been shown to affect different process, such as uncontrolled cell proliferation & differentiation and dysregulations in apoptosis, in the oncogenic process of MPM. It is important to mention that asbestos fibers have been related with increased prevalence of aberrant promoter methylation by controlling the APC and RASSF1 genes, directly affecting the cell cycle [1–4].

Epigenetic modifications require active maintenance and are potentially reversible, characteristics that make them targets for therapeutic strategies. Multiple DNA methyltransferases and histone deacetylases (HDACs) participate on the regulation of some tumor suppressor genes by gene silencing and chromatin compaction. Therefore, changes in these two enzymes promote disturbances in gene expression and allow deflections in cell proliferation, differentiation, and apoptosis. When HDACs are inhibited, there is a massive production of superoxide radicals and the caspase system is activated, leading to cell death. Additionally, hyperacetylation of non-histone proteins takes place, promoting angiogenesis and tumor cells motility and invasion [12].

DNA modifications are not the only mechanisms involved in tumorogenesis. Epigenetic changes also play an important role in oncogenesis through changes in DNA-associated proteins, modifying their expression. In this regard, the most important changes are DNA methylation and histone deacetylation. These changes lead to important modifications in DNA activity and expression. As a result of this process, some proteins involved in tumorogenesis can be induced and modulated, for example, epidermal growth receptor factor, tumor necrosis factor-alpha protein fusion peptide, transforming growth factor-beta and others. As mentioned above, these changes are induced by epigenetic mechanisms that are potentially reversible [12, 13].

In recent years, inhibiting tyrosinase-like receptors (RTKs) has been used as a therapeutic target because MPM cells have been shown to express high levels of receptors that can bind to key molecules, such as epidermal growth receptor factor (EGFR) and platelet-derived growth factor (PDGF), fibroblast growth receptor factor (FGFR-1y3), transforming growth factor-beta (TGF-B), insulin-like growth factor (IGF-1R), and tumor necrosis factor-alpha protein fusion peptide (NGR-hTNF-alpha). All these molecules undergo through epigenetic changes and play a dead serious role in tumor invasion and angiogenesis [12, 13].

Numerous genes have been shown to be epigenetically downregulated, as the DNA methylation of transcriptional promoters. These changes deregulate several signaling pathways, including the WNT pathway, in which several negative regulators are hypermethylated and silenced [14, 15]. The global epigenetic profile determined by high-throughput analysis differs between MPM and normal pleura, showing that MPM has aberrant methylation in the CpG islands, as has been mentioned [16, 17]. These data support the hypothesis that a specific DNA methylation pathway is induced during mesothelial carcinogenesis.

Kim et al. [1] carried out a study in a patient with MPM, 122 differently regulated genes were found, 118 genes were down-regulated and four were up-regulated by hypomethylation. Therefore, MPM cells may be epigenetically regulated, and DNA methylation plays a main role in intratumorally heterogeneity, characteristic that boost MPM more aggressiveness.

2.2 Factors associated with methylation

There are sundry important factors that have been related with DNA methylation of gene loci in MPM such as age-related changes, ethnicity, histological subtype, and asbestos exposure. These factors could explain discrepancies between DNA methylation frequencies in published studies, as well as the experimental method used to detect it. In patients diagnosed with MPM, an increased DNA methylation associated with increased age has been reported. Some studies have shown that methylation status of the IGFBP2 (insulin growth factor binding protein) locus and GDF10 (bone morphogenetic protein) locus is significantly higher in MPM in Japanese patients compared with US patients [18, 19].

There are some concrete characteristics that are related to specific genes, for example; RASSF1 suppressor gene has been reported to have a significantly higher frequency of aberrant methylation in epithelioid MPM than in the sarcomatoid subtype [20, 21]. Methylation of MT2A gene, is shown to differ between these two histological subtypes. Epithelioid and sarcomatoid mesotheliomas also have different methylation changes at 87 CpG islands [22, 23]. MT1A and MT2A gene loci associated with DNA methylation have also been described in MPM.

CpG island methylation in the CCND2, CDKN2A, CDKN2B, HPPBP1, and RASSF1 genes has been studied in correlation with asbestos exposure. The RASSF1 DNA methylation locus is related with a higher number of asbestos bodies in the lung. There are different methylation profiles in MPM according with its exposure to asbestos and a positive association between asbestos fiber load and CDKN2A, CDKN2B, RASSF1 methylation status, and MT1A at another 100 loci.

2.3 Methylation and diagnosis through DNA

Some differences have been described in DNA methylation for sundry genes between MPM, lung adenocarcinoma, and in non-malignant lung tissues. That's why, at these days, DNA methylation is an important tool in the diagnosis of MPM [20, 24]. Thus, the DNA methylation profile has potential helpfulness in the diagnostic of MPM and reject of other differential diagnoses. It has been demonstrated by high-throughput analyses for methylation, spanning several thousand CpG islands. It was recently suggested that DNA methylation at three specific loci: TMEM30B, KAZALD1, and MAPK13, could be useful in the differential diagnosis of MPM. In the near future, MPM diagnosis may be based on the methylation profile, but by now, further studies in larger populations are necessary before using a limited number of hypermethylated loci [19–21].

Other studies have shown alterations in the methylation status of individual genes, such as those HIC1, PYCARD, LZTS1, and SLC6A20. All of these genes have been associated with a good or bad prognosis [22, 23]. Besides, patients with MPM and a low frequency of DNA methylation had longer survival [22–24].

In view of the aberrant epigenetic events observed in MPM and the clinical value of histone deacetylase inhibitors (HDACis), the latter is currently being studied as a potential diagnostic method. However, insufficient data is yet available on the regulation of histone modifications, despite their crucial role in maintaining chromatin stability. These data are needed to support clinical trials based on HDACis [6, 7, 25, 26].

2.4 Epigenetic regulation in mesothelioma gene expression

Each nucleosome is made up of 147 base pairs (bp) of DNA wrapped twice around a histone octamer. Epigenetic regulation of gene expression occurs in the context of chromatin, the basic unit of the nucleosome. Lysine-rich histone tails extend from the nucleosome and provide sites for covalent and reversible binding, promoting processes such as acetylation, methylation, ubiquitination, phosphorylation and SUMOylation, which produce the activation or inhibition of gene expression [8, 27].

DNA methylations represent the most important mechanism regulating major changes in gene expression during normal cell cycle and tissue differentiation, as well as long-term repression of imprinted alleles, germ cell-restricted genes, repetitive DNA, and sequences. Endogenous retrovirals [27–29]. Normal somatic cells have three major DNA methyltransferases: DNMT1, DNMT3A, and DNMT3B. All these enzymes mediate the transfer of a methyl group from S-adenosyl-methionine to the 5′ position of cytosine in the context of CpG. CpG dinucleotide groups are found in the promoters of approximately 60% of genes. Furthermore, most of these islands are unmethylated, allowing for a relaxed structure (euchromatin) and active transcription [30]. Some other CpG dinucleotides and CpG islands, which are often hypermethylated in normal cells, are scattered throughout the genome [31]. Although there is considerable overlap, DNMT1 preferentially binds hypermethylated DNA and works primarily as a housekeeping methyltransferase, restoring DNA methylation patterns during the process of DNA repair or replication. On the other hand, DNMT3A and 3B mediate de novo DNA methylation after recognition of unmethylated or hypermethylated DNA [30, 31].

It is important to recapitulate that methylation-sensitive transcription factor binding is inhibited by DNA methylation, and these changes promote the recruitment of the CpG methyl-binding domain (MBD) and relevant proteins such as UHRF1, syn3a-containing repressor complexes, NCoRs and histone deacetylases (HDACs), resulting in silent transcriptional heterochromatin output [32–34].

During the process of malignant transformation, the aberrant orientation and overexpression of some factors involved in DNA methylation promote the epigenetic silencing of genes related to differentiation, many of which are tumor suppressors. On the other hand, tumor suppressor genes can be inactivated by DNA methylation through transitional mutations resulting from deamination of 5-methylcytosine (5-MC) or adduct formation with environmental carcinogens such as benzopyrene [35].

DNA demethylation occurs passively during DNA replication [36, 37]. In addition, DNA can be actively demethylated by oxidation of 5-MC to 5-hydroxymethylcytosine, a ten-eleven translocation (TET) enzyme-mediated reaction [20].

The total amount of methylated CpGs, during malignant transformation, is up to 50%, excluding CpG promoter islands. The genome-wide DNA demethylation is importantly related to a deficient DNA repair process [38–41]. Besides, it can promote unrepression of imprinted alleles, endogenous retroviruses, and transposable elements, inducing genomic instability [42, 43]. On the other hand, the mechanisms that mediate this phenomenon, such as decreased expression of methyltransferase 1 [44–46] glycosylase-mediated cleavage of 5-MC and aberrant expression/orientation of TET proteins, have not been fully elucidated [38].

The most widely characterized histone modifications in normal cells and malignant cells have been the acetylation-deacetylation and the methylation-demethylation [1, 2, 43, 47]. Histone acetylation is mediated by a variety of histone acetyltransferases (HAT), increasing the net negative charge leading to DNA repulsion, chromatin relaxation, and gene expression. Some non-histone proteins, including Hsp90, SP1, p53, and HDAC1, are targets for HAT and HDAC. In the other hand, histone deacetylation is regulated by HDAC [48].

Histone lysine methylation is mediated by a variety of histone methyltransferases (KMTs), lysine mediating monomethylation/dimethylation/trimethylation of specific residues, whereas histone demethylation is mediated by histone demethylases [47, 49, 50]. Histone modifications are highly dynamic in response to environmental signals [51, 52]. Unlike histone acetylation, histone lysine methylation does not modify the charge of core histones. Furthermore, histone lysine methylation can promote or inhibit gene expression.

ATP-dependent chromatin remodeling complexes have emerged, in recent years, as critical mediators of the epigenetic regulation of gene expression in normal and malignant cells [53, 54]. To date, four gene families have been described including switch/non-fermentable sucrose (SWI/SNF), SWI mimetic (ISWI), DNA-binding helicase chromodomain (CHD), and INO80, named for their ability to regulate inositol-responsive gene expression. All these complexes have multiple subunits with diverse isoforms and exhibit pleiotropic functions including regulation of gene expression, maintenance of chromatin structure, replication of pericentromeric heterochromatin, repression of ribosomal RNA, and repair of cell damage. DNA [55]. There are several mechanisms by which different families remodel chromatin. For example, the SWI/SNF complexes expose DNA by disassembling the nucleosome, while members of the ISWI, INO80, and CDH families reposition (slide) the nucleosomes and extend the intervening DNA, promoting access to transcriptional factors. These complexes also have an important role in maintaining chromatin structure and genome stability, through mechanisms that reassemble the nucleosome [53, 55].

Studies in transcriptome analysis have revealed that almost 90% of the genome is transcribed as non-coding RNAs (IncRNAs), which are critical mediators of chromatin structure and gene expression in normal cells and malignant transformation [56–58]. Besides, lncRNAs participate in the recruitment of DNMTs and histone methyltransferases to chromatin [59], adding another layer of epigenetic regulation in normal cells which is altered in malignant tumors.

3. Methylation-mediated suppressor gene silencing

There are several studies that have shown a relationship between silencing suppressor gene by methylation process and the development of MPL. For example, Christensen et al. [23] examined the DNA methylation status of the promoter of six genes that regulate cell cycle progression at 70 MPM. The extent of methylation of these genes was correlated with lung asbestos burden and overall survival. Goto et al. [60] studied methylation process in more than 6000 GpC islands, comparing twenty MPM versus twenty lung adenocarcinomas, using microarray PCR technique. Their results are interesting because they found out that 387 genes (6.3%) were hypermethylated in mesotheliomas, while the number of hypermethylated gene in lung adenocarcinoma were higher with a total amount of 544 genes (8.8%).

MPL patients' survival is related with DNA methylation levels. In this way, higher levels of DNA methylation correlate with lower patient survival. Three genes; TMEM30B, KAZALD1 and MAPK13, are specifically hypermethylated in MPM. Several reports have documented tumor suppressor gene silencing related to DNA methylation process in MPM (**Table 1**) and there is evidence of hypermethylation of some of these genes affecting overall survival.

Currently, scientific evidence has shown that recurrent hypermethylation is highly related to tumor suppressor genes in MPM, however, the mechanisms behind this process have been poorly studied. Novel studies have identified TC2N gene as a tumorigenesis promoter by silencing p53. Cytokine signaling participate in modulation process of DNMT expression and mediate hypermethylation of target genes enrolled in some types of cancer such as colorectal carcinoma and erythroleukemia cells [61, 62]. Exposure to asbestos fibers leads to a cytokine cascade induced by high mobility group 1 (HMGB1) or the NLRP3 inflammasome. These cytokines use to change the regulation of the expression of DNMT and other components of the methylation machinery during the process of MPM evolution.

A study of a panel of genes encoding epigenetic regulators in a panel of cultured cell lines derived from asbestos-associated MPM relative to LP-9 (a commercially available normal mesothelial cell line) was recently carried out. Consistent with the study results, TCGA data demonstrate a spectrum of DNMT expression in MPM and suggest that overexpression of DNMT1, DNMT3A, and DNMT3B correlates with decreased survival of pleural mesothelioma patients (**Figure 2**).

APC1A	P151NK4B
APC1B	P16
BMP3b	RARB
CDH1	RASSF1A
DAPK	SFRPs
ESR1	SLC6A20
FHIT	SYK
IGFBP3	TMEM30B
KAZALD1	THBD
MAPK13	TMEM30B
MGMT	TYMP
P14ARF	WIF-1

MPM: malignant pleural mesothelioma.

Table 1.
Hypermethylated genes related to MPM.

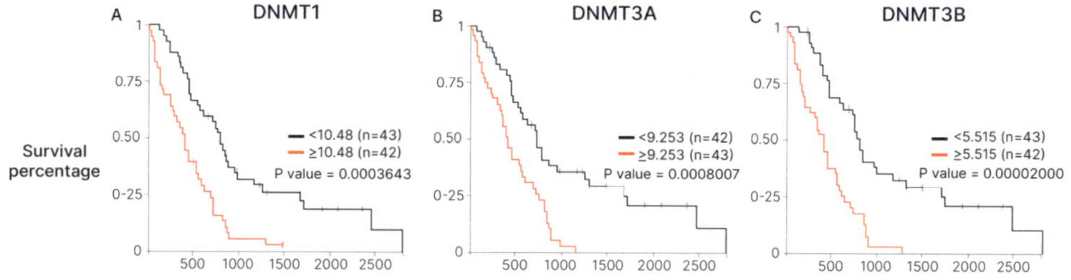

Figure 2.
Association between intratumoral DNMT expression levels and surveillance in patients with MPM. The Kaplan Meier waves show that DNMT1, DNMT3A, and DNMT3B expression, measured by RNA-seq technique, has negative impact in patients' surveillance.

Kim et al. [1] studied gene expression and methylation profiles in pluripotent populations (SP) and non-SP fractions in human MPM samples, using RNA-seq and methylated DNA immunoprecipitation techniques. They found 6400 hypermethylated genes and 3400 hypomethylated genes in SP. Seven hundred and ninety-five genes were upregulated, while three hundred and thirty-five were significantly repressed in SP compared to non-SP fractions. They looked at changes in DNA methylation and expression levels of 122 genes; 118 genes were hypermethylated and downregulated, while 4 were hypomethylated and upregulated. Ten other genes showed hypermethylation and low expression of CpG promoter islands.

4. Loss of imprinting (LI) and de-repression of cancer-germline (CG) genes

The loss of the imprinting process is largely due to DNA hypomethylation. Repression of endogenous retroviral sequences and activation of GC genes can promote malignant transformation by increasing proliferation, genomic instability, and resistance to apoptosis [63, 64].

A fascinating phenomenon can occur during the malignant transformation of somatic cells. The development of highly limited tumor antigens that induce serological and cell-mediated immune responses in cancer patients can be caused by abnormal activation of GC genes [also known as testicular cancer (TC) genes]. As a result, testicular cancer antigens (ATCs) have become popular targets for cancer immunotherapy in recent years [65]. More than 270 GC genes have been registered in the international TC database thus far. Seventy-five percent of these genes are only expressed in normal testes and malignant neoplasms, while the rest have high levels of expression in testes and varying levels of expression in other normal tissues and malignancies. On the X chromosome, around half of the GC genes are encoded. Families of cancer-testis-X (CT-X) chromosomal genes with inverted DNA repeats are common. On the other hand, inverted repetitive DNA sequences or extended families or are not linked to non-X CT genes [66, 67]. Furthermore, CT-X genes are frequently active in malignancies, and genes from families are increased in a tumor-specific manner, implying that the CT-X genes have a transcriptional coregulation and functional link.

In human malignancies, the stage at which the disease is discovered at a specific time corresponds to the degree of CG gene repression. Malignant and aggressive phenotype of cancer cells is promoted activations of this genes. BORIS/CTCFL, for example, upregulates h-TERT and suppresses apoptosis in cancer cells via processes that are still unknown [68, 69]. MAGE-A11 regulates the activity of the tumor suppressor gene RBL1/p107 [63]. MAGE-A11 inhibits the tumor suppressor gene RBL1/p107, while MAGE-B2 promotes cell cycle advancement by increasing E2F activity. MAGE-A2 and MAGE-C2 prevent p53 from binding to target promoters, changing its activities and leading to p53 deacetylation (inactivation) or enhanced ubiquitin-mediated degradation. The absence of CG gene regulation does not appear to be just a symptom of pluripotency, as it is accompanied with chromosomal hypomethylation. In human ESC, mesenchymal stem cells, and adipose-derived stem cells, Loriot et al. [70] found no overexpression of 18 different CG genes. In induced pluripotent stem cells (iPSCs) produced from normal small airway epithelial cells, transcriptional repression of CG genes such as NY-ESO-1, MAGE-A1, and MAGE-A3, which are generally located upward in thoracic malignant tumors, has been detected, which is consistent with these findings. Although these findings imply that iPSC reprogramming is partial, induction of CG genes in cancer cells may necessitate more extensive DNA hypomethylation as well as activation of tissue-specific transcription factors.

There is currently such little information on the expression of CG genes in MPM. MAGE1--4, NY-ESO-1, GAGE1-2, GAGE1-6, SSX2, SSX1-6, and RAGE-1 expression in five MPM lines was compared to normal mesothelial cells employing RT-PCR techniques, according to Sigalotti et al. [71]. In these MPM lines, diverse expressions of the CG gene were identified, with each line exhibiting a unique profile, as previously reported for lung malignancies [72]. None of these genes were found in normal mesothelial cells [71, 73].

5. Polycom complex-mediated epigenetic silencing

Polycomb group proteins (PcG) play an important role as regulators of stem cell pluripotency and differentiation [74], as well as inappropriate gene expression during cancer transformation [75, 76]. In mammals, two main Polycomb repressor complexes (PRCs) have been discovered. PRC-2 is an initiating complex that causes trimethylation of histone 3 lysine and contains the subunits EZH1/EZH2, SUZ12, EED, and RBAP46/48 (H3K27Me3).

PCAF, PHC, RING1, CBX, and BMI1 are components of the housekeeping complex PRC-1, which mediates the ubiquitination of H2AK119 (H2AK119Ub). CRC recruitment and heterochromatin growth are aided by these histone marks, which are frequently detected in the context of DNA hypermethylation and gene suppression [75, 76]. Several proteins, such as including JARID2 and members of the sex comb-like family (ASXL), interact with EZH2 and SUZ12 to lead PRC-2 to polykyl response elements (PRE) throughout the genome [77, 78]. Goto et al. [79] investigated gene repression in MPM and observed that a subset of genes repressed in MPM had H3K27Me3 without DNA hypermethylation, implying that disruptions in polycomb gene expression may play a role in MPM etiology [80, 81].

Several immunoblotting investigations studies revealed that MPM cells overexpress EZH2 with associated increases in H3K27Me3 levels when compared to normal mesothelial cells. Another set of tests, which included QRT-PCR, immunoblotting, and IHC, revealed that EZH2 was overexpressed in almost 80% of primary MPMs (most of which were epithelioid histology). As a result of these findings, it was identified that EZH2 is overexpressed in MPM and that PRC-2 could be considered as a potential therapeutic target in these cancers. The overexpression of EZH2 in MPM was verified by TCGA analysis, as was a strong link between EZH2 upregulation and lower MPM patient survival (**Figure 2A**). Further TCGA analysis reveals that SUZ12 overexpression is associated with poor survival in MPM patients (**Figure 2B**). On the other hand, there is no evidence about MPM patients' survival related to EED expression (**Figure 2C**).

The foregoing findings are especially important in light of recent findings that inactivating mutations in BRCA-associated protein 1 (BAP1), which encodes a nuclear ubiquitin hydrolase with several functions, are found in uncommon familial MPMs as well as almost 60% of sporadic MPMs. H2AK119Ub is ubiquitinated, for example.

LaFave et al. [82] discovered that BAP1 mutations, which are linked to protein expression loss, enhanced the expression of EZH2 and SUZ12 in MPM cells in a series of experiments. Likewise, overexpression of EZH2 was related to lower levels of H4K2Me1 and less occupancy of L3MBTL2 (an unusual polycomb protein that identifies this repressive histone mark) inside the EZH2 promoter in BAP1 mutant cells. Despite the strong connection between BAP1 mutations and repression of Polycomb stem cell targets, no specific clinical manifestation of BAP1 mutant MPM has been identified. Somatic mutations in BAP1 appear to be more common in current or past smokers with MPM [83].

6. SWI/SNF

SWI/SNF are mammalian homologs of yeast trithorax complexes. Their major purpose is to antagonize PRC-2's repressive effects by destroying DNA-nucleosome connections allowing movement and ejection, or by switching nucleosomes to increase factor accessibility transcription to DNA [84, 85]. In human malignancies, the genes encoding the SWI/SNF complexes are commonly altered, with various subunit mutations related to specific cancer histologies.

Yoshikawa et al. [86] used whole exome sequencing to identify a substantial number of mutations in genes involved in the SWI/SNF pathways, including homozygous SMARCA4, ARID2, and PBRM1 mutations in short-term established MPM lines [86, 87]. They also evaluated at the loss of somatic copies in the 3p21 region (which is roughly 10.7 Mb in size and contains 251 genes) in 33 MPM samples, using techniques including comparative genomic matrix high-density hybridization (a-CGH) and next-generation targeted sequencing (NGS). Bi-allelic deletions (3 Kb) were observed in 46 genes, four of which have been associated to malignant tumors, including two SWI/SNF-related genes [PBRM1 (15%) and SMARCC1 (6%)], BAP1 (48%) and SETD2 (27%). More than 200 MPM were studied in a recent thorough genomic investigation.

Bueno et al. [88] described mutations in genes encoding SWI/SNF components in 8% of the samples, as well as mutations in two histone methyltransferases (SETDB1 and SETD5) in about 3% of the samples. The discrepancies between the results reported by Yoshikawa et al. [87] and Bueno et al. [88] may be attributable to the identification of minuscule deletions by high-density, a-CGH, and specific NGS that are not detectable by conventional NGS techniques. To establish final conclusions, more studies are needed to determine the frequency and clinical significance of SWI/SNF mutations in mesothelioma.

7. Epigenetics in the treatment of mesothelioma

MPM inhibits tumor suppressor genes by promoting LOI and repression of CG genes by site-specific hypermethylation of DNA and/or polycomb repressor complexes in the context of hypomethylation of the genome. This "DNA methylation paradox" mimics epigenomic conditions in normal germ cells and lays the groundwork for epigenetic regimens that restore tumor suppressor gene expression and trigger growth arrest/apoptosis. Upregulation of CTAs, development of viral mimicry by derepression of endogenous retroviruses, and control of the tumor microenvironment all help to boost antitumor immunity [89, 90].

DNMTs are potential targets for MPM treatment because of their direct functions in suppressing tumor suppressor genes and maintaining pluripotency [91, 92]. Previous clinical attempts to inhibit DNMT activity in MPM, however, have failed miserably. Yogelzang et al. [93] showed a 17% objective response rate in 41 MPM patients who received 120 h of continuous dihydro-5-azacytidine infusions. Amazingly, 6 years following treatment, the single responder was disease-free. The lack of efficacy of DNA hypomethylating drugs in solid tumors could be due to their usage at maximum tolerated doses, resulting in myelosuppression, rather than prolonged use at lower doses to obtain pharmacodynamic effects without systemic toxicity. The Phase I decitabine trial (DAC) clearly demonstrates that chronic exposures are required to achieve maximum gene induction effects in cancer tissues [94].

Furthermore, 5-AZA and DAC administered IV, SQ, or PO have short half-lives (less than 5 min) and poor biodistribution, limiting their potential utility in patients with solid tumors. Cytidine deaminase (CDA), which is found in practically all organs but mainly the gastrointestinal system, quickly inactivates these molecules [95, 96]. Documented toxicity increases Cmax and t1/2 (>50 nM and 4 h, respectively) as well as biodistribution of oral decitabine, decreasing inter-patient variability in drug levels significantly [95–98]. Significant increases in fetal hemoglobin, without neutropenia, thrombocytopenia, or lymphopenia, are indicative of hypomethylation of systemic DNA caused by oral DAC-THU. A phase II trial (NCT02664181) is currently underway at the Cleveland Clinic and NCI to examine whether DAC/THU can improve responses to nivolumab when given as second-line therapy to patients with non-small cell lung cancer. Despite encouraging preclinical data [26], efforts to target HDAC on MPM have also been disappointing.

As second- or third-line therapy, Krug et al. [99] randomized 661 MPM patients to receive the HDAC inhibitor vorinostat or placebo. Overall survival, as well as the drug's safety and tolerability, were the key outcomes. Vorinostat-treated patients had a median OS of 30.7 weeks (95% CI 26.7–36.1) compared to 27 weeks (95% CI 23.1–31.9) for placebo-treated patients. Given the absence of evidence for HDAC upregulation in MPM and the limited antitumor effects of HDAC inhibitors alone in preclinical tests, the lack of efficacy of the single-agent vorinostat in patients with MPM is not surprising. Combinated techniques, such as using HDAC inhibitors to sensitize cells to TRAIL-mediated apoptosis or flavopiridol to boost romidepsin-mediated growth arrest and death, might be helpful for future clinical trials. Hypomethylating drugs, on the other hand, do not appear to lessen the incidence of mesothelioma after asbestos exposure. In fact, non-solid cancers such leukemias, lymphomas, and other myelodysplastic syndromes show the best benefits with this medicine.

It is feasible that BAP1 mutations could be used for MPM therapy in the future. BAP1 promotes the recruitment of the polychial deubiquitinase PR-DUB complex to

DNA damage sites by stabilizing BRCA-1 and promoting poly (ADP-Ribose) dependent recruitment of the polychial deubiquitinase PR-DUB complex to DNA damage sites. This activity is dependent on deubiquitinase activity and BAP1 phosphorylation. BAP1 mutations, which invariably show as a loss of function, cause BRCA-1 levels to drop and double-stranded DNA repair to be inhibited [100–102]. A BAP1 isoform including part of the catalytic domain sensitized MPM cells to the PARP1 inhibitor, according to Parotta et al. [102]. (Olaparib). Concomitant treatment with GDC0980, a dual PI3K-mTOR inhibitor that is downregulated by BRCA-1, could improve this sensitivity. These strategies could improve responses to cisplatin/pemetrexed in patients with BAP1 mutant MPM and should be evaluated in future clinical trials.

There is considerable interest in chromatographic remodeling agents with adoptive cell transfer or immune checkpoint inhibitors for cancer therapy, given the extensive preclinical studies showing DNA demethylating agents, HDAC inhibitors, and KMT inhibitors in the immunomodulatory effects of potentials [103]. In a syngeneic mouse tumor model, cytolytic T lymphocytes target testicular cancer antigen in vivo using decitabine to destroy metastatic cancer. The preclinical basis for combining gene induction regimens with cancer adoptive immunotherapy was established in these studies. Furthermore, novel microenvironmental data are likely to have a substantial impact on the outcomes of clinical trials for epigenetic treatments and immunotherapies [89].

8. Conclusions

While malignant pleural mesothelioma is a disease with a low incidence worldwide, with aggressive behavior, its survival does not go beyond 12 months once the diagnosis is made [1, 2]. Its origin has been related to the chronic exposure of asbestos as the main factor. Also, asbestos fibers have been an essential component in structural changes at the molecular level, with much evidence about its genetic behavior and to a lesser extent, its epigenetic behavior. All of this gives it a fairly heterogeneous behavior [13–15]. New molecular techniques allow a broader understanding of the carcinogenesis of this tumor and an approach to new diagnostic tools. Epigenetic dysregulations require active maintenance and are potentially reversible, making them a therapeutic target [7, 23, 30].

The study of methylome has made it possible to carry out differential diagnoses thanks to the methylation of some specific loci, such as TMEM30B, KAZAZD1, MAPK13 and to demonstrate greater survival rates in patients with low frequencies of methylations [16, 17, 28].

It is important to mention the exposure to asbestos fibers as the main resistance factor associated with the methylation of tumor suppressor genes seen in pleural mesothelial cells such as APC and RASSF1. Additionally, there are direct cellular effects such as chronic inflammation measured by free radicals leading to DNA oxidation, hemolysis with the release of hydroxyl ions, intrachain breakdown plus subsequent chromosomal fragmentation, and production of pro-inflammatory cytokines with higher expression of angiogenic growth factors, another aspect that can be considered a potential therapeutic objective. Genomic responses related to methylation conclude in a gene silencing, most likely in tumor suppressor genes such as SFRP4, FHIT, SLCA20 [69, 71, 80]. Another diagnostic approach that can be observed by methylation is the overexpression of DNMT in patients with MPM and consequently could be an attractive therapeutic target, however, clinical efforts for its inhibition have been disappointing and future studies should focus on the therapeutic approach to the inhibition of DNMT.

A greater association of methylation has been seen in advanced ages and ethnic groups such as the Japanese population. However, the greater association related to histological changes in proliferation, differentiation, invasion, and reduction of apoptosis has been seen with the increased methylation of CpG islands in genes such as CCND2, CDKN2A, and associated with asbestos bodies with RASSF1.

Although methylation is the most studied epigenetic mechanism, there are other modifications that lead to the silencing of tumor suppressor genes, such as the activation of the Polycomb complex and the mutation of the SWI/SNF pathway [82, 83]. Deacetylation mediated by HDAC has been seen in the p53 gene and other aspects such as HAT-mediated acetylation or demethylation by KDMs.

The modification in histone features such as stability in chromatin has a great relationship with HDCAs, thus making them a potential therapeutic target. There are few studies with inhibitors such as vorinostat, however, where there are no positive results due to the low expression in MPM.

Finally, it is clear that there is much to know about the modifications and/or epigenetic changes in MPM. The current evidence of the molecular mechanisms opens up another panorama for us to adjust personalized therapeutic strategies aimed at reversing normal changes and thus be able to identify in a timely manner those patients who are susceptible to such treatments. Therefore, clinical trials should focus on those epigenetic markers that at some point in their disease are overexpressed or silenced.

Author details

Aldo Manuel Alvarez Moran*, Pablo Alejandro Ávila Sánchez,
Jorge Alejandro Torres Ríos and Lorena Vega Castillo
The Anáhuac Puebla University School of Medicine, Puebla, Puebla, Mexico

*Address all correspondence to: mdald73@hotmail.com

References

[1] Kim MC, Kim NY, Seo YR, Kim Y. An integrated analysis of the genome-wide profiles of DNA methylation and mRNA expression defining the side population of a human malignant mesothelioma cell line. Journal of Cancer. 2016;**7**(12):1668-1679

[2] Sage AP, Martinez VD, Minatel BC, et al. Genomics and epigenetics of malignant mesothelioma. High-Throughput. 2018;**7**(20):2-23

[3] Feinberg AP, Ohlsson R, Henikoff S. The epigenetic progenitor origin of human cancer. Nature Reviews Genetics. 2006;**7**:21-33

[4] Magee JA, Piskounova E, Morrison SJ. Cancer stem cells: Impact, heterogeneity, and uncertainty. Cancer Cell. 2012;**21**:283-296

[5] Pietras A. Cancer stem cells in tumor heterogeneity. Advances in Cancer Research. 2011;**112**:255-282

[6] Sekido Y. Molecular pathogenesis of malignant mesothelioma. Carcinogenesis. 2013;**34**(7):1413-1419

[7] Heintz NH et al. Asbestos, lung cancers, and mesotheliomas: From molecular approaches to targeting tumor survival pathways. American Journal of Respiratory Cell and Molecular Biology. 2010;**42**:133-139

[8] Toyokuni S. Mechanisms of asbestos-induced carcinogenesis. Nagoya Journal of Medical Science. 2009;**71**(1-2):1-10

[9] Laird PW. Principles and challenges of genome-wide DNA methylation analysis. Nature Reviews Genetics. 2010;**11**:191-203

[10] Jacinto FV, Ballestar E, Esteller M. Methyl-DNA immunoprecipitation (MeDIP): Hunting down the DNA methylome. BioTechniques. 2008;**44**:35

[11] Blayney JK, Ceresoli GL, Castagneto B, O'Brien ME, Hasan B, et al. Response to chemotherapy is predictive in relation to longer overall survival in an individual patient combined-analysis with pleural mesothelioma. European Journal of Cancer. 2010;**48**:2983-2992

[12] Vandermeers F, Neelature Sriramareddy S, Costa C, Hubaux R, Cosse JP, et al. The role of epigenetics in malignant pleural mesothelioma. Lung Cancer. 2013;**81**:311-318

[13] Shukla A, Shukla A. Current therapies for malignant mesothelioma. Journal of Cancer Science and Therapy. 2014;**6**:306-309

[14] Lee AY, He B, You L, et al. Expression of the secreted frizzled-related protein gene family is downregulated in human mesothelioma. Oncogene. 2004;**23**(39):6672-6676

[15] Kohno H, Amatya VJ, Takeshima Y, et al. Aberrant promoter methylation of WIF-1 and SFRP1, 2, 4 genes in mesothelioma. Oncology Reports. 2010;**24**(2):423-431

[16] Christensen BC, Houseman EA, Godleski JJ, et al. Epigenetic profiles distinguish pleural mesothelioma from normal pleura and predict lung asbestos burden and clinical outcome. Cancer Research. 2009;**69**(1):227-234

[17] Goto Y, Shinjo K, Kondo Y, et al. Epigenetic profiles distinguish malignantpleural mesothelioma from lung adenocarcinoma. Cancer Research. 2009;**69**(23):9073-9082

[18] Tomii K, Tsukuda K, Toyooka S, et al. Aberrant promoter methylation of insulin-like growth factor binding protein-3 gene in human cancers. International Journal of Cancer. 2007;**120**(3):566-573

[19] Kimura K, Toyooka S, Tsukuda K, et al. The aberrant promoter methylation of BMP3b and BMP6 in malignant pleural mesotheliomas. Oncology Reports. 2008;**20**(5):1265-1268

[20] Toyooka S, Pass HI, Shivapurkar N, et al. Aberrant methylation and simian virus 40 tag sequences in malignant mesothelioma. Cancer Research. 2001;**61**(15):5727-5730

[21] Shivapurkar N, Toyooka S, Toyooka KO, et al. Aberrant methylation of trail decoy receptor genes is frequent in multiple tumor types. International Journal of Cancer. 2004;**109**(5):786-792

[22] Tsou JA, Galler JS, Wali A, et al. DNA methylation profile of 28 potential marker loci in malignant mesothelioma. Lung Cancer. 2007;**58**(2):220-230

[23] Christensen BC, Marsit CJ, Houseman EA, et al. Differentiation of lung adenocarcinoma, pleural mesothelioma, and nonmalignant pulmonary tissues using DNA methylation profiles. Cancer Research. 2009;**69**(15):6315-6321

[24] Tsou JA, Shen LY, Siegmund KD, et al. Distinct DNA methylation profiles in malignant mesothelioma, lung adenocarcinoma, and non-tumor lung. Lung Cancer. 2005;**47**(2):193-204

[25] Suzuki M, Toyooka S, Shivapurkar N, et al. Aberrant methylation profile of human malignant mesotheliomas and its relationship to SV40 infection. Oncogene. 2005;**24**(7):1302-1308

[26] Paik PK, Krug LM. Histone deacetylase inhibitors in malignant pleural mesothelioma: Preclinical rationale and clinical trials. Journal of Thoracic Oncology. 2010;**5**(2):275-279

[27] Dawson MA, Kouzarides T. Cancer epigenetics: From mechanism to therapy. Cell. 2012;**150**(1):12-27

[28] Tessarz P, Kouzarides T. Histone core modifications regulating nucleosome structure and dynamics. Nature Reviews. Molecular Cell Biology. 2014;**15**:703-708

[29] Jin B, Robertson KD. DNA methyltransferases, DNA damage repair, and cancer. Advances in Experimental Medicine and Biology. 2013;**754**:3-29

[30] Baylin SB, Jones PA. Epigenetic determinants of cancer. Cold Spring Harbor Perspectives in Biology. 2016;**8**(9):a019505

[31] Pruitt K. Molecular and cellular changes during cancer progression resulting from genetic and epigenetic alterations. Progress in Molecular Biology and Translational Science. 2016;**144**:3-47

[32] Yin Y, Morgunova E, Jolma A, et al. Impact of cytosine methylation on DNA binding specificities of human transcription factors. Science. 2017;**356**:eaaj2239

[33] Zhu H, Wang G, Qian J. Transcription factors as readers and effectors of DNA methylation. Nature Reviews. Genetics. 2016;**17**(9):551-565

[34] Shimbo T, Wade PA. Proteins that read DNA methylation. Advances in Experimental Medicine and Biology. 2016;**945**:303-320

[35] Yoon JH, Smith LE, Feng Z, et al. Methylated CpG dinucleotides are the preferential targets for G-to-T

transversion mutations induced by benzo[a]pyrene diol epoxide in mammalian cells: Similarities with the p53 mutation spectrum in smoking-associated lung cancers. Cancer Research. 2001;**61**(19):7110-7117

[36] Bochtler M, Kolano A, Xu GL. DNA demethylation pathways: Additional players and regulators. BioEssays. 2017;**39**:1-13

[37] Yin X, Xu Y. Structure and function of TET enzymes. Advances in Experimental Medicine and Biology. 2016;**945**:275-302

[38] An J, Rao A, Ko M. TET family dioxygenases and DNA demethylation in stem cells and cancers. Experimental & Molecular Medicine. 2017;**49**:323

[39] Zoghbi HY, Beaudet AL. Epigenetics and human disease. Cold Spring Harbor Perspectives in Biology. 2016;**8**(2):a019497

[40] Schomacher L, Niehrs C. DNA repair and erasure of 5-methylcytosine in vertebrates. BioEssays. 2017;**39**(3)

[41] Schuermann D, Weber AR, Schar P. Active DNA demethylation by DNA repair: Facts and uncertainties. DNA Repair (Amst). 2016;**44**:92-102

[42] Van Tongelen A, Loriot A, De Smet C. Oncogenic roles of DNA hypomethylation through the activation of cancer-germline genes. Cancer Letters. 2017;**396**:130-137

[43] Audia JE, Campbell RM. Histone modifications and cancer. Cold Spring Harbor Perspectives in Biology. 2016;**8**(4):a019521

[44] Ha K, Lee GE, Palii SS, et al. Rapid and transient recruitment of DNMT1 to DNA double-strand breaks is mediated by its interaction with multiple components of the DNA damage response machinery. Human Molecular Genetics. 2011;**20**:126-140

[45] Cai Y, Tsai HC, Yen RC, et al. Critical threshold levels of DNA methyltransferase 1 are required to maintain DNA methylation across the genome in human cancer cells. Genome Research. 2017;**27**:533-544

[46] Bagwe AN, Kay PH, Spagnolo DV. Evidence that DNA methylation imbalance is not involved in the development of malignant mesothelioma. Anticancer Research. 1997;**17**(5A):3341-3343

[47] Zhao Y, Garcia BA. Comprehensive catalog of currently documented histone modifications. Cold Spring Harbor Perspectives in Biology. 2015;7(9):a025064

[48] Wapenaar H, Dekker FJ. Histone acetyltransferases: Challenges in targeting bi-substrate enzymes. Clinical Epigenetics. 2016;**8**:59

[49] Hyun K, Jeon J, Park K, et al. Writing, erasing and reading histone lysine methylations. Experimental & Molecular Medicine. 2017;**49**:e324

[50] Yi X, Jiang XJ, Li XY, et al. Histone methyltransferases: Novel targets for tumor and developmental defects. American Journal of Translational Research. 2015;7:2159-2175

[51] Filipp FV. Crosstalk between epigenetics and metabolism-Yin and Yang of histone demethylases and methyltransferases in cancer. Briefings in Functional Genomics. 2017;**16**(6):320-325

[52] Liu F, Killian JK, Yang M, et al. Epigenomic alterations and gene expression profiles in respiratory epithelia exposed to cigarette

smoke condensate. Oncogene. 2010;**29**:3650-3664

[53] Kumar R, Li DQ, Muller S, et al. Epigenomic regulation of oncogenesis by chromatin remodeling. Oncogene. 2016;**35**:4423-4436

[54] Längst G, Manelyte L. Chromatin remodelers: From function to dysfunction. Genes (Basel). 2015;**6**(2):299-324

[55] Thapa B, Salcedo A, Lin X, et al. The immune microenvironment, genome-wide copy number aberrations, and survival in mesothelioma. Journal of Thoracic Oncology. 2017;**12**:850-859

[56] Rinn JL, Chang HY. Genome regulation by long noncoding RNAs. Annual Review of Biochemistry. 2012;**81**:145-166

[57] Rinn JL. lncRNAs: Linking RNA to chromatin. Cold Spring Harbor Perspectives in Biology. 2014;**6**(8):a018614

[58] Meseure D, Drak Alsibai K, Nicolas A, et al. Long noncoding RNAs as new architects in cancer epigenetics, prognostic biomarkers, and potential therapeutic targets. BioMed Research International. 2015;**2015**:320214

[59] Davidovich C, Cech TR. The recruitment of chromatin modifiers by long noncoding RNAs: Lessons from PRC2. RNA. 2015;**21**(12):2007-2022

[60] Goto Y, Shinjo K, Kondo Y, et al. Epigenetic profiles distinguish malignant pleural mesothelioma from lung adenocarcinoma. Cancer Research. 2009;**69**:9073-9082

[61] Foran E, Garrity-Park MM, Mureau C, et al. Upregulation of DNA methyltransferase-mediated gene silencing, anchorage-independent growth, and migration of colon cancer cells by interleukin-6. Molecular Cancer Research. 2010;**8**:471-481

[62] Qureshi MA, Khan S, Tauheed MS, et al. Pan-cancer multiomics analysis of TC2N gene suggests its important Role(s) in tumourigenesis of many cancers. Asian Pacific Journal of Cancer Prevention. 2020;**21**(11):3199-3209

[63] Gaudet F, Hodgson JG, Eden A, et al. Induction of tumors in mice by genomic hypomethylation. Science. 2003;**300**:489-492

[64] Salmaninejad A, Zamani MR, Pourvahedi M, et al. Cancer/testis antigens: Expression, regulation, tumor invasion, and use in immunotherapy of cancers. Immunological Investigations. 2016;**45**:619-640

[65] De Smet C, Loriot A. DNA hypomethylation and activation of germline-specific genes in cancer. Advances in Experimental Medicine and Biology. 2013;**754**:149-166

[66] Simpson AJ, Caballero OL, Jungbluth A, et al. Cancer/testis antigens, gametogenesis and cancer. Nature Reviews. Cancer. 2005;**5**:615-625

[67] Zendman AJ, Ruiter DJ, Van Muijen GN. Cancer/testis-associated genes: Identification, expression profile, and putative function. Journal of Cellular Physiology. 2003;**194**(3):272-288

[68] Renaud S, Loukinov D, Alberti L, et al. BORIS/CTCFL-mediated transcriptional regulation of the hTERT telomerase gene in testicular and ovarian tumor cells. Nucleic Acids Research. 2011;**39**:862-873

[69] Zhou J, Cheng T, Li X, et al. Epigenetic imprinting alterations as

effective diagnostic biomarkers for early-stage lung cancer and small pulmonary nodules. Clin. Epigenetics. 2021;**13**(1):220

[70] Loriot A, Reister S, Parvizi GK, et al. DNA methylation-associated repression of cancer-germline genes in human embryonic and adult stem cells. Stem Cells. 2009;**27**:822-824

[71] Sigalotti L, Coral S, Altomonte M, et al. Cancer testis antigens expression in mesothelioma: Role of DNA methylation and bioimmunotherapeutic implications. British Journal of Cancer. 2002;**86**:979-982

[72] Schrump DS. Targeting epigenetic mediators of gene expression in thoracic malignancies. Biochimica et Biophysica Acta. 2012;**1819**(7):836-845

[73] Weiser TS, Guo ZS, Ohnmacht GA, et al. Sequential 5-Aza-2 deoxycytidine-depsipeptide FR901228 treatment induces apoptosis preferentially in cancer cells and facilitates their recognition by cytolytic T lymphocytes specific for NY-ESO-1. Journal of Immunotherapy. 2001;**24**:151-161

[74] Oliviero G, Brien GL, Waston A, et al. Dynamic protein interactions of the polycomb repressive complex 2 during differentiation of pluripotent cells. Molecular & Cellular Proteomics. 2016;**15**:3450-3460

[75] Pasini D, Di Croce L. Emerging roles for Polycomb proteins in cancer. Current Opinion in Genetics & Development. 2016;**36**:50-58

[76] Poynter ST, Kadoch C. Polycomb and trithorax opposition in development and disease. Wiley Interdisciplinary Reviews: Developmental Biology. 2016;**5**(6):659-688

[77] Pasini D, Cloos PA, Walfridsson J, et al. JARID2 regulates binding of the Polycomb repressive complex 2 to target genes in ES cells. Nature. 2010;**464**:306-310

[78] Katoh M. Functional proteomics of the epigenetic regulators ASXL1, ASXL2 and ASXL3: A convergence of proteomics and epigenetics for translational medicine. Expert Review of Proteomics. 2015;**12**(3):317-328

[79] Mantsoki A, Devailly G, Joshi A. CpG island erosion, polycomb occupancy and sequence motif enrichment at bivalent promoters in mammalian embryonic stem cells. Scientific Reports. 2015;**5**:16791

[80] Harikumar A, Meshorer E. Chromatin remodeling and bivalent histone modifications in embryonic stem cells. EMBO Reports. 2015;**16**(12):1609-1619

[81] Kemp CD, Rao M, Xi S, et al. Polycomb repressor complex-2 is a novel target for mesothelioma therapy. Clinical Cancer Research. 2012;**18**:77-90

[82] LaFave LM, Beguelin W, Koche R, et al. Loss of BAP1 function leads to EZH2-dependent transformation. Nature Medicine. 2015;**21**:1344-1349

[83] Zauderer MG, Bott M, McMillan R, et al. Clinical characteristics of patients with malignant pleural mesothelioma harboring somatic BAP1 mutations. Journal of Thoracic Oncology. 2013;**8**:1430-1433

[84] Kadoch C, Copeland RA, Keilhack H. PRC2 and SWI/SNF chromatin remodeling complexes in health and disease. Biochemistry. 2016;**55**(11):1600-1614

[85] Pulice JL, Kadoch C. Composition and function of mammalian SWI/SNF chromatin remodeling complexes in human disease. Cold Spring Harbor Symposia on Quantitative Biology. 2016;**81**:53-60

[86] Yoshikawa Y, Sato A, Tsujimura T, et al. Biallelic germline and somatic mutations in malignant mesothelioma: Multiple mutations in transcription regulators including mSWI/SNF genes. International Journal of Cancer. 2015;**136**:560-571

[87] Yoshikawa Y, Emi M, Hashimoto-Tamaoki T, et al. High-density array-CGH with targeted NGS unmask multiple noncontiguous minute deletions on chromosome 3p21 in mesothelioma. Proceedings of the National Academy of Sciences of the United States of America. 2016;**113**:13432-13437

[88] Bueno R, Stawiski EW, Goldstein LD, et al. Comprehensive genomic analysis of malignant pleural mesothelioma identifies recurrent mutations, gene fusions and splicing alterations. Nature Genetics. 2016;**48**:407-416

[89] Wolff F, Leisch M, Greil R, et al. The double-edged sword of (re)expression of genes by hypomethylating agents: From viral mimicry to exploitation as priming agents for targeted immune checkpoint modulation. Cell Communication and Signaling: CCS. 2017;**15**:13

[90] Kim K, Skora AD, Li Z, et al. Eradication of metastatic mouse cancers resistant to immune checkpoint blockade by suppression of myeloid-derived cells. Proceedings of the National Academy of Sciences of the United States of America. 2014;**111**:11774-11779

[91] Pathania R, Ramachandran S, Elangovan S, et al. DNMT1 365 is essential for mammary and cancer stem cell maintenance and tumorigenesis. Nature Communications. 2015;**6**:6910

[92] Yang J, Corsello TR, Ma Y. Stem cell gene SALL4 suppresses transcription through recruitment of DNA methyltransferases. The Journal of Biological Chemistry. 2012;**287**(3):1996-2005

[93] Yogelzang NJ, Herndon JE 2nd, Cirrincione C, et al. Dihydro-5-azacytidine in malignant mesothelioma. A phase II trial demonstrating activity accompanied by cardiac toxicity. Cancer and Leukemia Group B Cancer. 1997;**79**:2237-2242

[94] Schrump DS, Fischette MR, Nguyen DM, et al. Phase I study of decitabine-mediated gene expression in patients with cancers involving the lungs, esophagus, or pleura. Clinical Cancer Research. 2006;**12**:5777-5785

[95] Chabner BA, Johns DG, Coleman CN, et al. Purification and properties of cytidine deaminase from normal and leukemic granulocytes. The Journal of Clinical Investigation. 1974;**53**:922-931

[96] Lavelle D, Vaitkus K, Ling Y, et al. Effects of tetrahydrouridine on pharmacokinetics and pharmacodynamics of oral decitabine. Blood. 2012;**119**:1240-1247

[97] Wentworth DF, Wolfenden R. On the interaction of 3,4,5,6-tetrahydrouridine with human liver cytidine deaminase. Biochemistry. 1975;**14**(23):5099-5105

[98] Newman EM, Morgan RJ, Kummar S, et al. A phase I, pharmacokinetic, and pharmacodynamic evaluation of the DNA methyltransferase inhibitor 5-fluoro-2′-deoxycytidine, administered with tetrahydrouridine. Cancer

Chemotherapy and Pharmacology. 2015;**75**:537-546

[99] Krug LM, Kindler HL, Calvert H, et al. Vorinostat in patients with advanced malignant pleural mesothelioma who have progressed on previous chemotherapy (VANTAGE-014): A phase 3, double-blind, randomised, placebo-controlled trial. The Lancet Oncology. 2015;**16**:447-456

[100] Ismail IH, Davidson R, Gagne JP, et al. Germline mutations in BAP1 impair its function in DNA double-strand break repair. Cancer Research. 2014;**74**:4282-4294

[101] Fukuda T, Tsuruga T, Kuroda T, et al. Functional link between BRCA1 and BAP1 through histone H2A, heterochromatin and DNA damage response. Current Cancer Drug Targets. 2016;**16**:101-109

[102] Yu H, Pak H, Hammond-Martel I, et al. Tumor suppressor and deubiquitinase BAP1 promotes DNA double-strand break repair. Proceedings of the National Academy of Sciences of the United States of America. 2014;**111**:285-290

[103] Parrotta R, Okonska A, Ronner M, et al. A novel BRCA1-associated protein-1 isoform affects response of mesothelioma cells to drugs impairing BRCA1-mediated DNA repair. Journal of Thoracic Oncology. 2017;**12**(8):1309-1319

Section 2

Diagnostic Aspects of Mesothelioma

Chapter 3

Mesothelioma: Overview of Technical, Immunochemical and Pathomorphological Diagnosing Aspects

Ave Minajeva and Diana Saranova

Abstract

For the clinicians with non-pathology background, first encountering the patients with pleural or peritoneal effusions, mesothelioma is only one statistically rare but clinically significant option of many differential diagnoses. This review aims to help the clinicians and broad life science audiences to understand step by step the possibilities and shortcomings of pathological diagnosing of mesothelioma, including the basic technical requirements. The first cytomorphology evaluation of pleural and peritoneal effusions in routinely stained smears enables in most cases only to identify cells suspicious for malignancy. The recent guidelines of epithelioid mesothelioma cytologic diagnosis and reporting emphasize immunochemistry (IC) in the cell blocks is mandatory whenever a diagnosis of malignancy is clinically entertained and/or cytologically suspected. The IC workup is challenging, since there is no fixed antibody panel, but multiple questions must be solved, such as 1) confirm the mesothelial or epithelial origin of isolated atypical cells and cell clusters; 2) delineate their benign or malignant nature; and 3) discriminate mesothelioma from other malignancics and metastatic disease. The rationale of the most widely clinically used IC markers is given and illustrated by the examples. The final confirmation of mesothelioma diagnosis and establishing its subtype and grade is possible only in the histological samples.

Keywords: mesothelioma, carcinoma, effusion, immunochemistry, cell block, cytology, histology

1. Introduction

Mesothelioma is a rare and malignant tumor arising from the mesothelial or submesothelial cells of the pleura, peritoneum, or pericardium. Until 2021, the term "malignant" had been used as a prefix for mesothelioma in order to distinguish it from the well-differentiated papillary mesothelioma. In the recently updated WHO Classification, this was renamed well-differentiated papillary mesothelial tumor (WDPMT), to highlight its differences from diffuse mesothelioma, the word "malignant" has been dropped [1]. Mesothelial tumor diagnoses according to the 2021 WHO Classification of

Benign and pre-invasive mesothelial tumors
Adenomatoid tumor
Well-differentiated papillary mesothelial tumor
Mesothelioma in situ
Mesothelioma
Localized mesothelioma
Diffuse mesothelioma
Epithelioid mesothelioma
Sarcomatoid mesothelioma
Mesothelioma, biphasic

Table 1.
Mesothelial tumors.

the tumors of the pleura and pericardium are summarized in **Table 1**. If not otherwise stated, most cases of mesothelioma in the literature refer to diffuse mesothelioma. There are rare benign mesothelial tumors such as adenomatoid tumor and WDPMT, only the latter will be briefly discussed in this review. Mesothelioma in situ refers to a flat noninvasive form of mesothelioma and localized mesothelioma is histologically identical to diffuse, but macroscopically solitary, circumscribed mass. Both of these are very rare, only a very few cases have been described [2, 3].

More than 80% of all diffuse mesotheliomas originate in the pleura and 10–15% are peritoneal [4, 5]. Clinical manifestations of mesothelioma are usually nonspecific and, due to a broad spectrum of differential options, can be difficult to diagnose especially in the early stage. The diagnosis of mesothelioma has to be made in the context of appropriate clinical, radiologic, and surgical findings. Because patients with mesotheliomas frequently present with effusions, sampling of pleural or peritoneal fluid for biochemical and cytological examination is often the first source of material [6–8]. The sampled diagnostic material bears limitations in pathological analysis. As cytological smear alone is insufficient for diagnosing mesothelioma, the utilization of immunochemistry (IC) must be applied to confirm both the mesothelial origin and its malignant nature, and exclude other potential mimickers such as metastatic carcinomas [8–11]. Final confirmation of the diagnosis and establishing the histological type, grade, and invasiveness of mesothelioma can be done in biopsy or operation material. Mesotheliomas are histologically divided into epithelioid, sarcomatoid, and biphasic varieties.

Current review aims to highlight the basic steps of the pleural and peritoneal mesothelioma pathological diagnosis along with most important technical handling details for clinicians and broad life science audiences. The sample figures of cytological and histological findings are from the archives of the North Estonian Medical Centre, the identity of patients remains unrevealed and the ethics committee permission is, therefore, unrequired.

2. Effusion fluid as a first-hand cytologic diagnostic material

2.1 Clinical conditions of differential significance

Mesothelioma is often but not always represented with effusion, the sampled fluid is typically exudate, yellowish, and often bloody [12]. It is reported to be thick and mucoid owing to hyaluronic acid or hyaluronan content. Notably hyaluronan and

N-ERC/mesothelin increase in effusion fluid predict mesothelioma with high specificity, prior to pathological examination. Pleural CEA increase can rule out mesothelioma with a high degree of certainty. Other soluble mesothelioma biomarkers such as C-ERC/mesothelin, osteopontin, fibulin-3, syndecan-1, syndecan-2, and thioredoxin are lacking sufficient accuracy for clinical use [13–15].

The diagnostic difficulty arises since there is a large diversity of other diseases, which can manifest with pleural or peritoneal effusions, creating an abundance of differential diagnoses to navigate in the cytological study. From a pathologist's perspective, benign infective, inflammatory, or other diseases are causing reactive changes in the mesothelial cells. Such reactive conditions manifesting predominantly with exudation can be related to tuberculous pleuritis or empyema or parapneumonic effusion caused by other bacteria, and collagen vascular diseases. Additionally, effusion can also be transudative because of hypoalbuminemia and heart or renal failure [16]. Among benign conditions causing peritoneal exudative effusion are infections such as tuberculosis or spontaneous bacterial peritonitis, whereas predominantly transudative effusion or ascites can be caused by portal hypertension due to liver cirrhosis, alcoholic hepatitis, or hepatic congestion, but also pancreatitis, hypoalbuminemia, or renal failure [17]. Reactive mesothelial cell changes can be extremely hard to distinguish from malignancy (see later). Therefore, another crucial question pathologist face is to confirm malignancy in the effusion cytology and to differentiate mesothelioma from other malignancies such as lung cancer and pleural metastasis from other organs, especially the breast [16]. In peritoneal effusions, other malignancies except mesothelioma to bear in mind are primary peritoneal papillary serous carcinoma, but more often hepatocellular carcinoma, metastatic liver disease, lymphoma with peritoneal involvement or the spread of other intra-abdominal malignancies such as pancreatic, gastric, colorectal, ovarian, or renal carcinomas [17–19]. Pathological differential diagnosis can help to identify the primary site of malignancy in a patient with a history of multiple malignancies or an unknown primary site.

2.2 Handling of material

Accuracy of pathological diagnosis heavily relies on high quality of material, which depends on its proper handling. The removed effusion is preferably sent to the laboratory fresh if possible with anticoagulants (heparin ethylenediaminetetraacetic acid or sodium citrate) present, but without added fixatives, and it should be refrigerated at 4°C until processing. When longer transportation times are needed, a volume of 50% ethanol can be added as a preservative [9].

Upon arrival in the laboratory, the fluid should be processed without delay. Refrigerated samples should be brought to room temperature, particularly when using preparation techniques associated with liquid-based cytology (LBC). To prepare a cell pellet, the material is centrifuged at 1000 g or more for 10 min. For the cytomorphological evaluation, smears are prepared from centrifuged deposits (preferably by cytospin method) and routinely stained with one of the Giemsa modifications (Romanowsky-Giemsa, Leishman-Giemsa or May-Grünewald-Giemsa kits), which enables well to examine cytoplasmic characteristics. Many labs are splitting the sample and use also Papanicolaou (PAP) stain preferably in liquid-based cytology to facilitate for nuclear evaluation [20].

The recent guidelines of mesothelioma diagnosis require additional IC studies (see later), which can be applied on smears, but the most popular technique is the cell block, obtained after the sediments from cytological specimens are processed, formalin-fixed and embedded into paraffin blocks that can be serial sectioned and stained by the same methods used for histopathology [21].

3. Cytological diagnosis of mesothelioma

3.1 Cytological features of mesothelioma in routinely stained smears

Evaluating the cytomorphology of pleural and peritoneal effusions in routinely stained smears enables in most cases to identify malignant cells and suspicious for malignancy. In either case, to discriminate reactive proliferative mesothelium from mesothelioma and other malignancies, ancillary IC studies are required (see later). Some cases cannot be diagnosed by cytology like cases with minimal cell shedding, typically almost all sarcomatoid mesotheliomas. However, sarcomatoid mesothelioma can be overlaid by the reactive epithelioid mesothelial cells, which may readily shed into fluids and mislead the pathologist. Sarcomatoid mesothelioma can be successfully diagnosed only histologically by using core biopsy (or larger tissue samples) [21]. Since the cells in effusion are exfoliative from the tumor surface, and cytology material is lacking access to the deep structures, assessment of invasion of preexisting tissues and its correlation to the clinical and imaging findings are not possible.

Cytological features of mesothelioma are outlined in abundance for pathology specialists [9], but this information is based on histologically confirmed retrospective studies. There is significant overlap between mesothelioma, reactive mesothelial cells, and adenocarcinoma or anaplastic tumors [8, 22]. Also, a rare WDPMT has considerable cytological overlap with mesothelioma [23–25].

Figure 1 represents an example of the peritoneal fluid cytology with confirmed epithelioid mesothelioma by later histological studies. The basic general cytomorphological criteria indicating possible mesothelioma are: (1) material containing large numbers of mesothelial cells, including large ball-shaped or papillary cell aggregates with knobby outlines (scalloped borders) and (2) presence of overtly malignant cells, either as single cells or in tissue fragments [9].

The malignant mesothelial cells can be significantly larger than normal, and each of the components of the whole cell is enlarged: cytoplasm, nucleus, and nucleolus.

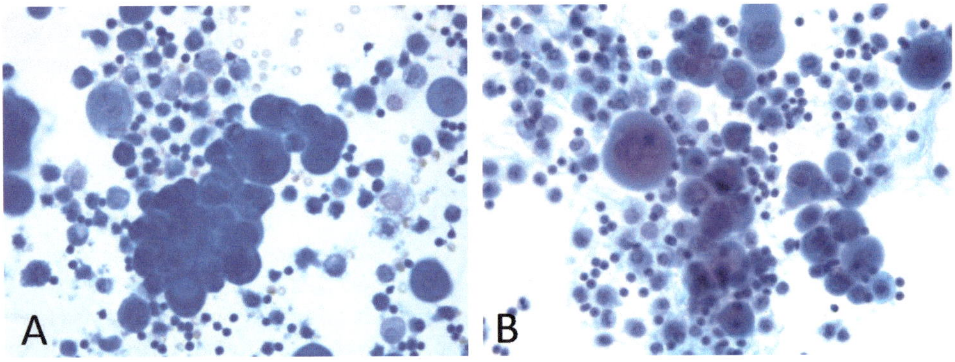

Figure 1.
Cytomorphology of the peritoneal epithelioid mesothelioma in effusion. Peritoneal effusion cytospin in epithelioid mesothelioma stained with Leishman-Giemsa (A) and Papanicolaou (PAP) stain (B), original magnification ×400. The specimen is highly cellular, containing large cell cluster (A) and papillary-shaped aggregates (B). Large mesothelial cells with macronucleoli and multinucleated cells (A and B).

The cells may be multinucleated, contain prominent macronucleoli or there are vacuoles overlapping with cell nuclei. Protrusions from the cell membrane or blebbing and prominent degree of cell-within-cell arrangements are also characteristics. Background may be acidophilic due to large amounts of hyaluronan and contain granular extracellular matrix fragments of collagen and basement membrane cores, as well as multinucleated giant cells and small pyknotic eosinophilic cells [9].

3.2 General aspects of immunochemistry

Effusion cytology work-up mostly faces discrimination of epithelioid mesothelioma since sarcomatoid subtype rarely exfoliates in the fluids. The recent guidelines of epithelioid mesothelioma cytologic diagnosis and reporting emphasize the role of IC in conjunction with the cytomorphologic evaluation because it substantially increases diagnostic accuracy [9, 21]. IC on cell blocks is mandatory whenever a diagnosis of malignancy is clinically entertained and/or cytologically suspected [21].

There is no fixed IC panel or absolute number of antibodies that can be recommended for the diagnosis of mesothelioma. Workup can be done in stages. It is recommended that a panel of at least four antibodies should be used, two in favor and two against mesothelioma. The diagnosis should never be based on one single IC reaction. Numerous antibodies for mesothelioma are commercially available, but most are not entirely specific and may show cross-reactivity with other tumors [9]. It has to be emphasized that only validated antibodies should be used for clinical diagnosis and different antibody clones have to be carefully tested with appropriate controls in the labs. If possible, antibodies should be chosen with a sensitivity or specificity of at least 80% [9]. The staining patterns (i.e., nuclear, cytoplasmic, and membranous) are important for most antibodies, and since these may differ with the new antibody clones, up-to-date information has to be followed and the tests performed with appropriate controls. There is no standard for the percentage of tumor cells that should be positive, but some have used a 10% cutoff for membranous and cytoplasmic staining [9]. IC results should be interpreted in complexity and in the context of morphological and clinical data. Of notice, the cell blocks can be also used for molecular studies, which is beyond the scope of this review.

3.3 Immunochemical workup of mesothelioma

The antibodies used for mesothelioma IC workup are largely similar in effusion cell blocks and in histological tissue blocks, however, some extra advice is added for antibody application in tissues.

The diagnosis in effusions is more challenging, comprising the following tasks: 1) confirm the mesothelial or epithelial origin of isolated atypical cells and cell clusters; 2) delineate their benign or malignant nature; and 3) discriminate mesothelioma from other malignancies and metastatic disease, which can show diffuse pleural or peritoneal spread.

Summary of the most widely clinically used IC markers will be given and illustrated by the examples in **Figure 2**. For the rest of markers, only brief references are given [8]. The paraffin-embedded cell blocks are sectioned and stained similarly to the histological specimen and, therefore, a routine hematoxylin and eosin (H&E) staining is also applied, which provides additional cytomorphological evaluation (**Figure 2A**).

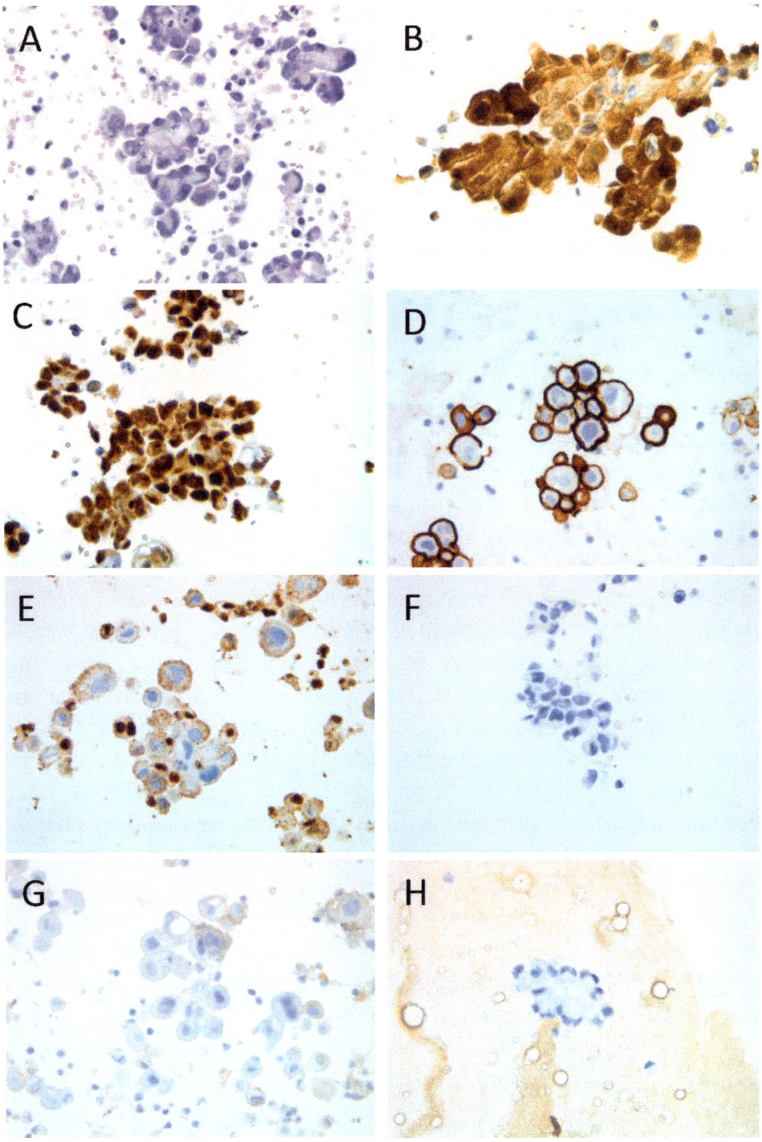

Figure 2.
Malignant mesothelioma in peritoneal fluid cytoblock. A staining panel confirming mesothelial origin, malignancy, and discriminating from gastrointestinal and gynecologic tumors. All antibodies are applied as ready-to-use (RTU) solutions, the producers are shown in the brackets. A, H&E stain to assess cytomorphology: Highly cellular specimen, enlarged atypical cell aggregates, with hyperchromatic pleomorphic nuclei and vacuolated cytoplasm could be seen (original magnification ×400). B, Calretinin expression both in nuclei and cytoplasm (Ventana, RTU, ×400). C, WT1 specific staining is nuclear (Ventana, RTU, ×400). D, D2–40 strong membranous expression (Dako, RTU, ×400). E, BAP-1 shows nuclear loss of expression in mesothelioma cells, whereas reactive mesothelial cells and background lymphocytes retain nuclear staining (BioSB, RTU, ×400). F, CEA negative (Dako, RTU, ×400). G, Ber-Ep4 negative with minimal nonspecific stain (Dako, RTU, ×400). H, CDX2 negative in mesothelioma cells (nonspecific background stain) (Dako, RTU, ×400).

3.3.1 Markers used to confirm mesothelial origin

Markers of mesothelial cells are immunoreactive with both benign and malignant cells.

3.3.1.1 Calretinin

The recent Calretinin antibodies (**Figure 2B**) require both nuclear and cytoplasmic staining to support a diagnosis of mesothelioma [26]. There are earlier reports of only nuclear staining with "fried egg appearance" [27, 28]. Cytoplasmic staining alone should be interpreted negatively [27]. In effusions, the sensitivity of calretinin in detecting mesothelioma ranges from 81 to 100% [26, 29, 30].

Calretinin can be expressed in breast carcinomas [31], and a weak cytoplasmic staining is reported in variety if other adenocarcinomas [27, 28]. Some studies have shown calretinin positivity in squamous cell carcinoma (SCC) of the lung ranging from 40 to 100% [27, 32].

3.3.1.2 Wilms tumor-1 (WT1)

Specific WT1 staining in mesothelioma is only nuclear (**Figure 2C**). WT1 frequently cross-reacts with cytoplasmic proteins in a variety of benign and malignant entities [33]. WT1 nuclear reactivity was reported in more than 90% of mesothelioma effusion specimens versus 20–30% of metastatic adenocarcinomas, particularly of pulmonary and breast origin [34–36]. In contrast, WT1 is not useful to distinguish peritoneal mesothelioma from ovarian/Mullerian tumors in effusions, since it is expressed in 80%–90% of ovarian malignancy [35, 37], and of notice, not recommended as a carcinoma-specific marker of these tumors either [8].

3.3.1.3 D2-40/podoplanin

D2–40 and podoplanin are specific lymphatic endothelial markers [38].

D2–40 immunostain shows strong membranous staining pattern in mesothelial cells (**Figure 2D**), with reported sensitivity of 83–100% and specificity of 49–100% [30, 39, 40].

Podoplanin has been shown to be even more specific than D2–40, but the number of studies is limited. Podoplanin is expressed in 94% of mesothelioma, 97% of reactive mesothelial cells, and 7% ovarian adenocarcinoma, while it is nonreactive in lung and breast adenocarcinoma, with an overall sensitivity and specificity of 94% and 97%, respectively, for mesothelioma [38]. While podoplanin showed strong membranous reactivity in mesothelioma cells, ovarian adenocarcinoma exhibited weak membranous staining [38].

3.3.2 Markers differentiating benign from malignant mesothelial proliferations

Many of the markers supposedly differentiating mesothelioma from benign reactive mesothelial cells have limited sensitivity or a too broad spectrum of reactivity. For example, relevance of EMA, p53, IMP-3, CD146, or glucose transporter 1 in defying benign and malignant cases is questioned, especially in histology materials [21].

3.3.2.1 BRCA1-associated protein (BAP1)

BAP1 is a nuclear ubiquitin hydrolase involved in various cellular processes, including chromatin remodeling. *BAP1* behaves as a true tumor suppressor gene.

BAP1 double-hit inactivation is a key driver event in about half of all mesotheliomas [41, 42]. Loss of BAP1 expression by IC can be a useful adjunct to distinguish mesothelioma from reactive mesothelial proliferations in some cases [43]. However, BAP1 is not very sensitive, with a reported loss of nuclear staining only in 27–57% of mesothelioma but in none of the reactive mesothelial cells [41, 42]. For correct interpretation, only nuclear loss of staining is accepted as true loss of expression [8]. Reactive mesothelial cells and background lymphocytes should express nuclear staining and can serve as internal control (**Figure 2E**).

BAP1 use has more limitations since it is preserved in many non-mesothelial malignancies, frequently encountered in effusion cytology, and BAP1 loss may be also encountered in other malignancies rarely seen in effusions such as malignant melanoma and urothelial carcinoma [44].

3.3.2.2 Enhancer of zeste 2 homolog (EZH2)

EZH2 is a member of the family of polycomb group genes (PcGs), which is a group of important epigenetic regulators that repress transcription. BAP1 loss can promote cell proliferation *in vitro* through up-regulation of EZH2 [45]. High EZH2 expression was observed in 66% of malignant mesothelioma cases, whereas none of the benign lesions showed high EZH2 expression. The combination of BAP1 loss and high EZH2 expression as markers to differentiate epithelioid/biphasic malignant mesothelioma from benign mesothelial lesions was highly sensitive (87–90%) and specific (100%) [46, 47]. Using IC alone for EZH2 also yielded a good sensitivity of 86.9%; this level is high enough for routine diagnostics [47].

3.3.2.3 Methylthioadenosine phosphorylase (MTAP)

MTAP is located in the 9p21.3 locus and is often deleted with p16. Detection of homozygous deletion of the 9p21.3 region by p16-fluorescence in situ hybridization is a reliable marker for malignancy in mesothelial effusions. MTAP IC has been suggested as a good surrogate marker for 9p21.3 deletion in surgical and cytology specimens [48]. The association of MTAP and BAP1 IC staining loss can reportedly detect mesothelioma with 78% sensitivity [49]. Only cytoplasmic loss of MTAP should be interpreted as a true loss of expression [48, 49].

3.3.2.4 Desmin

Since benign mesothelial cells express desmin, reactive proliferative mesothelial cells also express desmin in 84%–92% cases, whereas mesothelioma cells only in 0%–6% [30, 50]. Mesothelial cells tend to lose their cytoplasmic desmin expression as they transition to malignancy [22]. Attention has to be paid that any malignant effusion with mesothelioma still has few background reactive mesothelial cells which still are expressing desmin.

3.3.2.5 Epithelial membrane antigen (EMA)

EMA is expressed in adenocarcinoma with a very high sensitivity 91%–100% and a specificity of 86%–100% in differentiating adenocarcinoma from reactive mesothelial cells in effusions [51, 52]. EMA has distinctive staining of the cytoplasmic membrane brush border in mesothelioma, while it exhibits a diffuse cytoplasmic staining pattern in carcinomas [53].

3.3.3 Carcinoma markers

Due to close morphological resemblance, mesothelioma most often has to be differentiated from adenocarcinoma, but depending on location, many other types of carcinoma may be considered diagnostically important. The IC markers are serving two purposes: 1) distinguish broadly carcinoma cells from mesothelial malignancy and 2) differentiate carcinomas of a specific type or location.

3.3.3.1 Carcinoembryonic antigen (CEA)

CEA is a recommended marker for discriminating between mesothelioma and adenocarcinoma in effusions [54] (**Figure 2F**). It has a high reported specificity (90%–100%) and variable sensitivity (43%–100%) [54, 55] in detecting adenocarcinoma in effusions and exhibits a strong membranous staining pattern [55]. Monoclonal CEA antibody is more commonly used in effusions and generally preferred over polyclonal antibody to avoid the nonspecific staining in background inflammatory cells [8]. CEA is less specific in tissue sections as carcinomas of various origins and well-differentiated neuroendocrine tumors are negative with monoclonal CEA antibodies on tissue sections [56].

3.3.3.2 Claudin-4 (CL-4)

CL-4 belongs to a family of tight junction-associated proteins expressed in most epithelial cells but absent in mesothelial cells. CL-4 is a useful pan-carcinoma marker for serous effusion specimen, showing strong diffuse membranous expression pattern in 84%–96% adenocarcinomas and being negative in most mesotheliomas [57, 58]. CL-4 is useful also in tissue sections, where it has been expressed in 91% of carcinomas of different types and negative in mesothelioma [57]. CL-4 has a sensitivity of 85%–99% and specificity of 99%–100% in distinguishing carcinoma versus mesothelioma [57–61]. CL-4 is also very useful in detecting single tumor cells dispersed among heavy inflammatory reactions [61] or metastatic epithelial cells in serous effusions [8, 57, 61].

3.3.3.3 Ber-EP4

Ber-EP4 is an epithelial cell adhesion molecule (TACSTD1) that shows a predominantly membranous pattern [55]. Mesothelial cells are shown negative for Ber-EP4 in most studies (**Figure 2G**) [8]. Ber-EP4 has a sensitivity of 76%–94%, and specificity of 84%–100% in detecting adenocarcinoma [8, 51, 54, 55]. It is also reportedly positive in 87%–100% of SCC cases [8, 32].

3.3.4 Additional markers for organ/differentiation specific differentiation

In addition to general carcinoma markers, many antibodies can be helpful for detecting specific differentiation of cells and distinguishing mesothelioma from other malignancies in specific settings. **Table 2** summarizes some of their most common applications [7, 8, 62].

	Antibodies for organ-specific differentiation of mesothelioma
Lung adenocarcinoma	TTF1, Napsin A
Breast	GATA3, ER, PR, mammoglobin, GCDFP15
Thyroid	TTF1, Pax8, thyroglobulin
Squamous cell carcinoma	p40, p63, CK5/6
Renal cortical	Pax8, Pax2, CA9, RCC
Mullerian/ovarian origin	Pax8, Pax2, WT1, BerEP4, ER
Colorectal	SATB2, CDX2
Liver	HepPar1, Arginase-1, AFP
Prostate	NXK3.1, PSMA, PSA
Urotelial	p63, p40, GATA3
Malignant melanoma	SOX10, HMB45, S100, MART1, MITF
Hematopoietic	CD45, CD43, CD3, CD20, CD34, CD117, TdT

Table 2.
Additional immunostains used for organ-specific differentiation of epithelioid mesothelioma.

4. Histological sampling and typing of mesothelial tumors

4.1 General considerations of histological diagnostic material

Tissue sampling is currently achieved either by image-guided/thoracoscopic-guided or surgical biopsy, both of which are recommended by major guideline committees. Surgical biopsies in principle generate more tissue materials, occasionally as much as pleural decortication and extrapleural pneumonectomy.

Biopsies comprise too little tissue and are known to suffer from sampling bias. Microscopically, tissue fields from pleural and peritoneal cavities are often obscured by inflammation and fibrinous debris. Subpleural or intraperitoneal fat sampling, important in the assessment of invasion, may be absent in cases of significantly thickened pleura or peritoneum. False-positive immunostaining may be seen in tiny needle biopsy specimens with crushed artifacts and at the edges of biopsy samples [21].

Larger materials give better overview, especially of intra-tumoral heterogeneity and invasion, but to get these results, the materials should be sampled extensively. The histologic diagnosis should be based on both the appropriate morphology and on IC findings.

4.2 Well-differentiated papillary mesothelial tumor (WDPMT)

WDPMT is a relatively uncommon subtype of mesothelial neoplasm with a distinct molecular profile [63] and histological appearance [25, 64]. It arises most commonly in the peritoneal cavity, but can also be found in the pleural cavity, pericardium, and tunica vaginalis [25, 64, 65]. WDPMT typically exhibits indolent behavior and is generally considered of low malignant potential [64].

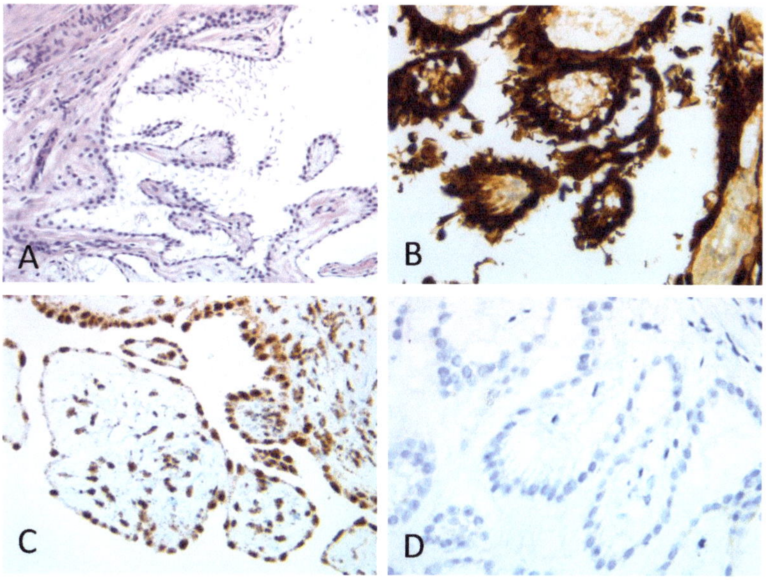

Figure 3.
Peritoneal well-differentiated papillary mesothelial tumor histology. A, H&E stain shows fibrovascular papillae lined by a simple uniform cuboidal epithelium, without nuclear atypia or mitoses (original magnification ×400). B, Calretinin expression both in nuclei and cytoplasm of lining epithelium confirms its mesothelial origin. The lining epithelial cell has enlarged appearance due to very intense staining (Ventana, RTU, ×400). C, BAP-1 expression is retained and shows uniform nuclear expression confirming benign nature of lining mesothelial cells (BioSB, RTU, ×400). D, PAX8 negativity helps to differentiate the serous neoplasms of ovaries and peritoneum (Abcam, 1:200, ×400).

Histologically, WDPMT usually has an architecture of fibrovascular papillae, lined by a simple uniform cuboidal epithelium, with little to no nuclear atypia or mitoses (**Figure 3A**). Areas of invasion are typically not seen [64, 66]. The lining epithelium bears immunochemical profile of mesothelium, showing nuclear and cytoplasmic positive expression of calretinin (**Figure 3B**). BAP-1 staining is particularly helpful as retained nuclear expression shows benign nature of lining epithelial cells (**Figure 3C**). Great care should be taken to differentiate WDPMP from serous neoplasms of the ovaries and peritoneum, where IC markers, for example PAX8, are highly useful (**Figure 3D**) [23].

4.3 Diffuse mesothelioma histological diagnosis

Examples of diffuse mesothelioma histological types are illustrated in **Figure 4**. Epithelioid mesothelioma comprises approximately 80% of all pleural mesotheliomas and is defined as being composed of epithelioid, rounded, or polygonal cells [1, 62, 67]. Epithelioid mesothelioma can have various architectural patterns depending if the cells are located in solid sheets or form tubular, papillary, adenomatoid, and trabecular patterns [62, 67]. Sarcomatoid mesothelioma is the second most common subtype, composed of elongated spindle cells arranged in solid sheets or within fibrous stroma [62, 67]. Biphasic mesotheliomas are composed of both epithelioid and sarcomatoid components and at least 10% of each component is required for definite diagnosis in resection specimen. Regardless if a diagnosis is made in biopsy or extended operation material, sarcomatoid components should be reported and quantified in the pathology report, because it influences the treatment and prognosis.

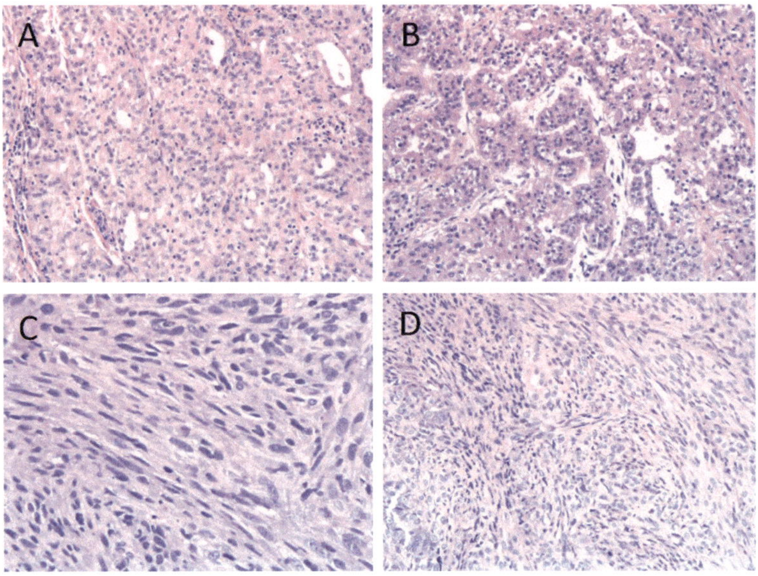

Figure 4.
Diffuse pleural mesothelioma histological subtypes. A, epithelioid mesothelioma is composed of rounded cells with eosinophilic cytoplasm and round nuclei with small nucleoli. In this tumor, the cells are located mostly in solid sheets with few gland-like structures (H&E stain, original magnification ×200). B, epithelioid mesothelioma architectural patterns may comprise trabecular, tubulopapillary, and gland-like structures (H&E, ×200). C, Sarcomatoid mesothelioma pattern is characterized by malignant elongated spindle-shaped cells (H&E, × 400). D, diffuse biphasic mesothelioma, which shows both epithelioid and sarcomatoid malignant areas (H&E, ×200).

IC is essential in establishing a diagnosis, and the choice of antibodies, particularly carcinoma markers, depends on histological architecture, and also whether the tumor has a pleural or peritoneal location. In pleural location, lung adenocarcinoma, SCC, and breast carcinomas are the most frequent differential diagnoses, but metastases from a variety of other organs could be confused with epithelioid mesothelioma. The case of pleural epithelioid mesothelioma presented in **Figure 5**, presence of psammoma bodies along with few papillary areas required an extended panel for testing ovarian serous carcinoma and gastrointestinal carcinomas (not shown), all of which were negative. Peritoneal mesotheliomas most often need to be distinguished from gastrointestinal, renal, and ovarian malignancies.

Epithelioid mesotheliomas are graded using a two-tiered system (low and high grade), combining nuclear grade (mitotic count and nuclear atypia) and presence of necrosis, because these features have been demonstrated to be strongly predictive of survival in patients with epithelioid mesothelioma [1, 62].

Sarcomatoid mesothelioma should be distinguished from metastatic sarcomatoid carcinomas from lung and other sites, particularly renal carcinomas [62]. Differential diagnosis can be challenging because markers can overlap, and will not be fully reviewed here. Immunochemical profile of sarcomatoid mesothelioma is different from the epithelioid. Sarcomatoid mesotheliomas are at least focally positive for cytokeratins AE1/AE, pan-cytokeratin (OSCAR), and anti-cytokeratin clone 1(KL1), as well as cytokeratin CAM5.2 [62, 68]. But sarcomatoid mesotheliomas can be cytokeratin-negative. Sarcomatoid mesotheliomas are positive for mesothelial

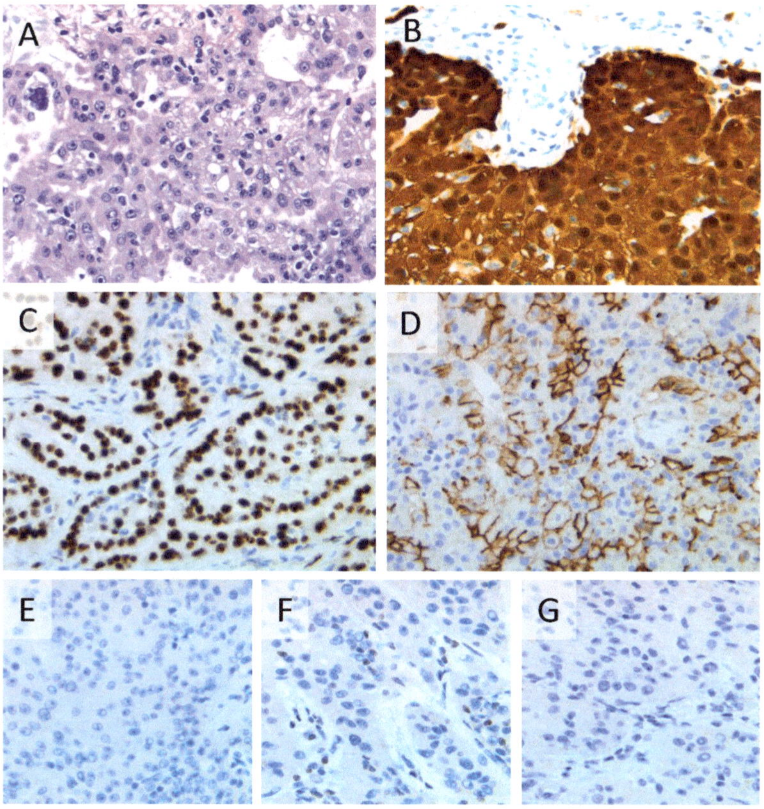

Figure 5.
Pleural epithelioid mesothelioma histology. A, H&E stain shows tubulopapillary mesothelioma structures. Tumor cells display moderate eosinophilic cytoplasm, mostly round nuclei with vesicular chromatin and small nucleoli. Psammoma body is seen in upper left corner (original magnification ×400). If concentrations are not indicated, antibodies are applied as ready-to-use (RTU) solutions. B, Calretinin diffuse expression both in nuclei and cytoplasm of malignant cells (Ventana, RTU, ×400). C, WT1 positive expression in all mesothelioma cell nuclei, but negative in fibrous stroma (Ventana, RTU, ×400). D, D2–40 strong membranous expression in most of the mesothelioma cells (Dako, RTU, ×400). E, TTF1 negativity in mesothelioma cells differentiates it from adenocarcinoma of the lung (Ventana, RTU, ×400). F, GATA3 negativity in mesothelioma cells differentiates it from breast carcinoma. Weak positivity is seen in the nuclei of lymphocytes (Ventana, RTU, ×400). G, PAX8 negativity in mesothelioma cells to differentiate from serous ovarian carcinoma (Abcam, 1:200, ×400).

markers such as calretinin, WT1, and D2–40 in limited cases [62, 68]. Sarcomatoid mesotheliomas are often vimentin-positive, whereas epithelioid mesotheliomas are often negative to vimentin. Occasionally, sarcomatoid mesotheliomas express actin, desmin, or S100 [62].

5. Conclusions

Diagnosing mesothelioma is a stepwise process, requiring complex orientation in a vast spectrum of clinical conditions and their corresponding pathological morphological criteria along with immunochemical proof. It needs careful individual decisions for applying ancillary studies and drawing proper conclusions considering the limitations of each diagnostic specimen.

Conflict of interest

The authors declare no conflict of interest.

Author details

Ave Minajeva[1*] and Diana Saranova[2]

1 Department of Pathological Anatomy and Forensic Medicine, University of Tartu, Institute of Biomedicine and Translational Medicine, Tartu, Estonia

2 Pathology Department of the North Estonia Medical Centre, Tallinn, Estonia

*Address all correspondence to: ave.minajeva@ut.ee

References

[1] Sauter JL, Dacic S, Galateau-Salle F, Attanoos RL, Butnor KJ, Churg A, et al. The 2021 WHO classification of tumors of the pleura: Advances since the 2015 classification. Journal of Thoracic Oncology. 2022;**17**(5):608-622

[2] Dacic S, de Perrot M, Gill RR, Hiroshima K, Klebe S, Nabeshima K. Mesothelioma in situ. In: Thoracic Tumours WHO, editor. Classification of Tumours. 5th ed. Lyon: WHO Classification of Tumours Editorial Board; 2021. pp. 200-201

[3] Khoor A, Bironzo P, Bueno R, Novak AKSF. Localized plaural masothelioma. In: Thoracic Tumours WHO, editor. Classification of Tumours. 5th ed. Lyon: WHO Classification of Tumours Editorial Board; 2021. pp. 202-203

[4] Moolgavkar SH, Meza R, Turim J. Pleural and peritoneal mesotheliomas in SEER: Age effects and temporal trends, 1973-2005. Cancer Causes & Control. 2009;**20**(6):935-944

[5] Teta MJ, Mink PJ, Lau E, Sceurman BK, Foster ED. US mesothelioma patterns 1973-2002: Indicators of change and insights into background rates. European Journal of Cancer Prevention. 2008;**17**(6):525-534

[6] Bibby AC, Tsim S, Kanellakis N, Ball H, Talbot DC, Blyth KG, et al. Malignant pleural mesothelioma: An update on investigation, diagnosis and treatment. European Respiratory Review. 2016;**25**(142):472-486

[7] Eccher A, Girolami I, Lucenteforte E, Troncone G, Scarpa A, Pantanowitz L. Diagnostic mesothelioma biomarkers in effusion cytology. Cancer Cytopathology. 2021;**129**(7):506-516

[8] Mneimneh WS, Jiang Y, Harbhajanka A, Michael CW. Immunochemistry in the work-up of mesothelioma and its differential diagnosis and mimickers. Diagnostic Cytopathology. 2021;**49**(5):582-595

[9] Hjerpe A, Ascoli V, Bedrossian C, Boon M, Creaney J, Davidson B, et al. Guidelines for cytopathologic diagnosis of epithelioid and mixed type malignant mesothelioma. Complementary statement from the international mesothelioma interest group, also endorsed by the international academy of cytology and the Papanicolaou society o. Cytojournal. 2015;**12**:26

[10] Pinto D, Chandra A, Crothers BA, Kurtycz DFI, Schmitt F. The international system for reporting serous fluid cytopathology—Diagnostic categories and clinical management. Journal of American Society Cytopathology. 2020;**9**(6):469-477

[11] Michael CWHK. In: Michael CWHK, Hjerpe A, Onal B, Segal A, editors. The International System for Reporting Serous Fluid Cytopathology. 1st ed. Switzerland AG: Springer Nature; 2020

[12] Ribak J, Lilis R, Suzuki Y, Penner L, Selikoff IJ. Malignant mesothelioma in a cohort of asbestos insulation workers: Clinical presentation, diagnosis, and causes of death. Occupational and Environmental Medicine. 1988;**45**(3):182-187

[13] Mundt F, Nilsonne G, Arslan S, Csürös K, Hillerdal G, Yildirim H, et al. Hyaluronan and N-ERC/Mesothelin as key biomarkers in a specific two-step model to predict pleural malignant mesothelioma. PLoS One. 2013;**8**(8):e72030

[14] Porcel JM. Biomarkers in the diagnosis of pleural diseases: A 2018 update. Therapeutic Advances in Respiratory Disease. 2018;**12**:175346661880866

[15] Saraya T, Ohkuma K, Fujiwara M, Ishii H. Diagnostic method for malignant pleural effusion distinguishing malignant mesothelioma from lung cancer using pleural carcinoembryonic antigen and hyaluronic acid levels. Medicine (Baltimore). 2022;**101**(1):e28517

[16] Light RW. Pleural Effusions. The Medical Clinics of North America. 2011;**95**(6):1055-1070

[17] Oey RC, van Buuren HR, de Man RA. The diagnostic work-up in patients with ascites: Current guidelines and future prospects. The Netherlands Journal of Medicine. 2016;**74**(8):330-335

[18] Di Muzio B, Stanislavsky A. Malignant peritoneal mesothelioma. In: Radiopaedia.org. Radiopaedia.org; 2010. DOI: 10.53347/rID-12677

[19] Bell D, Radswiki T. Primary peritoneal neoplasms. In: Radiopaedia.org. Radiopaedia.org; 2011. DOI: 10.53347/rID-14518

[20] Rao N, Wei S. Mesothelioma. Cytojournal. 2022;**19**:10. DOI: 10.25259/CMAS_02_08_2021. Available from: https://www.ncbi.nlm.nih.gov/pmc/articles/PMC9063505/

[21] Husain AN, Colby TV, Ordóñez NG, Allen TC, Attanoos RL, Beasley MB, et al. Guidelines for pathologic diagnosis of malignant mesothelioma 2017 update of the consensus statement from the international mesothelioma interest group. Archives of Pathology & Laboratory Medicine. 2018;**142**(1):89-108

[22] Hjerpe A, Ascoli V, Bedrossian CWM, Boon ME, Creaney J, Davidson B, et al. Guidelines for the Cytopathologic diagnosis of epithelioid and mixed-type malignant mesothelioma: A secondary publication. Cytopathology [Internet]. 2015;**26**(3):142-156 Available from:https://onlinelibrary.wiley.com/doi/10.1111/cyt.12250

[23] Nasit JG, Dhruva G. Well-differentiated papillary mesothelioma of the peritoneum. American Journal of Clinical Pathology. 2014;**142**(2):233-242

[24] Gong Y, Ren R, Ordóñez NG, Sun X, Sneige N. Fine needle aspiration cytology of well-differentiated papillary mesothelioma. Acta Cytologica. 2005;**49**(5):537-542

[25] Haba T, Wakasa K, Sasaki M. Well-differentiated papillary mesothelioma in the pelvic cavity. Acta Cytologica. 2003;**47**(1):88-92

[26] Shield PW, Koivurinne K. The value of calretinin and cytokeratin 56 as markers for mesothelioma in cell block preparations of serous effusions. Cytopathology. 2008;**19**(4):218-223

[27] Chhieng DC, Yee H, Schaefer D, Cangiarella JF, Jagirdar J, Chiriboga LA, et al. Calretinin staining pattern aids in the differentiation of mesothelioma from adenocarcinoma in serous effusions. Cancer. 2000;**90**(3):194-200

[28] Barberis MCP, Faleri M, Veronese S, Casadio C, Viale G. Calretinin. Acta Cytologica. 1997;**41**(6):1757-1761

[29] Fetsch PA, Simsir A, Brosky K, Abati A. Comparison of three commonly used cytologic preparations in effusion immunocytochemistry. Diagnostic Cytopathology. 2002;**26**(1):61-66

[30] Hyun TS, Barnes M, Tabatabai ZL. The diagnostic utility of D2-40, Calretinin, CK5/6, Desmin

and MOC-31 in the differentiation of mesothelioma from adenocarcinoma in pleural effusion cytology. Acta Cytologica. 2012;**56**(5):527-532

[31] Ordóñez NG, Sahin AA. Diagnostic utility of immunohistochemistry in distinguishing between epithelioid pleural mesotheliomas and breast carcinomas: A comparative study. Human Pathology. 2014;**45**(7):1529-1540

[32] Ordóñez NG. The diagnostic utility of immunohistochemistry in distinguishing between epithelioid mesotheliomas and squamous carcinomas of the lung: A comparative study. Modern Pathology. 2006;**19**(3):417-428

[33] Conner JR, Cibas ES, Hornick JL, Qian X. Wilms tumor 1/cytokeratin dual-color immunostaining reveals distinctive staining patterns in metastatic melanoma, metastatic carcinoma, and mesothelial cells in pleural fluids: An effective first-line test for the workup of malignant effusions. Cancer Cytopathology. 2014;**122**(8):586-595

[34] Hecht JL, Lee BH, Pinkus JL, Pinkus GS. The value of Wilms tumor susceptibility gene 1 in cytologic preparations as a marker for malignant mesothelioma. Cancer. 2002;**96**(2):105-109

[35] Pu RT, Pang Y, Michael CW. Utility of WT-1, p63, MOC31, mesothelin, and cytokeratin (K903 and CK5/6) immunostains in differentiating adenocarcinoma, squamous cell carcinoma, and malignant mesothelioma in effusions. Diagnostic Cytopathology. 2008;**36**(1):20-25

[36] Ordóñez NG. What are the current best immunohistochemical markers for the diagnosis of epithelioid mesothelioma? A review and update. Human Pathology. 2007;**38**(1):1-16

[37] Zhu W, Michael CW. WT1, monoclonal CEA, TTF1, and CA125 antibodies in the differential diagnosis of lung, breast, and ovarian adenocarcinomas in serous effusions. Diagnostic Cytopathology. 2007;**35**(6):370-375

[38] Hanna A, Pang Y, Bedrossian CWM, Dejmek A, Michael CW. Podoplanin is a useful marker for identifying mesothelioma in malignant effusions. Diagnostic Cytopathology. 2010;**38**(4): 264-269. DOI: 10.1002/dc.21340

[39] Bhalla R, Siddiqui MT, Mandich D, Cartun RW, Fiel-Gan MD, Nassar A, et al. Diagnostic utility of D2-40 and podoplanin in effusion cell blocks. Diagnostic Cytopathology. 2007;**35**(6):342-347

[40] Saad RS, Lindner JL, Lin X, Liu YL, Silverman JF. The diagnostic utility of D2-40 for malignant mesothelioma versus pulmonary carcinoma with pleural involvement. Diagnostic Cytopathology. 2006;**34**(12):801-806

[41] Andrici J, Sheen A, Sioson L, Wardell K, Clarkson A, Watson N, et al. Loss of expression of BAP1 is a useful adjunct, which strongly supports the diagnosis of mesothelioma in effusion cytology. Modern Pathology. 2015;**28**(10):1360-1368

[42] Sheffield BS, Hwang HC, Lee AF, Thompson K, Rodriguez S, Tse CH, et al. BAP1 immunohistochemistry and p16 FISH to separate benign from malignant mesothelial proliferations. The American Journal of Surgical Pathology. 2015;**39**(7):977-982

[43] Hiroshima K, Wu D, Hamakawa S, Tsuruoka S, Ozaki D, Orikasa H, et al. HEG1, BAP1, and MTAP are useful in cytologic diagnosis of malignant mesothelioma with effusion. Diagnostic Cytopathology. 2021;**49**(5):622-632

[44] Tesch ME, Pater JA, Vandekerkhove G, Wang G, Binnington K, So AI, et al. Concurrent germline and somatic pathogenic BAP1 variants in a patient with metastatic bladder cancer. Npj Genomic Medicine. 2020;**5**(1):12

[45] LaFave LM, Béguelin W, Koche R, Teater M, Spitzer B, Chramiec A, et al. Loss of BAP1 function leads to EZH2-dependent transformation. Nature Medicine. 2015;**21**(11):1344-1349

[46] Shinozaki-Ushiku A, Ushiku T, Morita S, Anraku M, Nakajima J, Fukayama M. Diagnostic utility of BAP1 and EZH2 expression in malignant mesothelioma. Histopathology. 2017;**70**(5):722-733

[47] Yoshimura M, Kinoshita Y, Hamasaki M, Matsumoto S, Hida T, Oda Y, et al. Highly expressed EZH2 in combination with BAP1 and MTAP loss, as detected by immunohistochemistry, is useful for differentiating malignant pleural mesothelioma from reactive mesothelial hyperplasia. Lung Cancer. 2019;**130**:187-193

[48] Hida T, Hamasaki M, Matsumoto S, Sato A, Tsujimura T, Kawahara K, et al. Immunohistochemical detection of MTAP and BAP1 protein loss for mesothelioma diagnosis: Comparison with 9p21 FISH and BAP1 immunohistochemistry. Lung Cancer. 2017;**104**:98-105

[49] Kinoshita Y, Hida T, Hamasaki M, Matsumoto S, Sato A, Tsujimura T, et al. A combination of MTAP and BAP1 immunohistochemistry in pleural effusion cytology for the diagnosis of mesothelioma. Cancer Cytopathology. 2018;**126**(1):54-63

[50] Hasteh F, Lin GY, Weidner N, Michael CW. The use of immunohistochemistry to distinguish reactive mesothelial cells from malignant mesothelioma in cytologic effusions. Cancer Cytopathology. 2010;**118**(2):90-96

[51] Stoop JA, Hendriks JGM, Berends D. Identification of malignant cells In serous effusions using a panel of monoclonal antibodies Ber-Ep4, Mca-B-12 and Ema. Cytopathology. 1992;**3**(5):297-302

[52] Murugan P, Siddaraju N, Habeebullah S, Basu D. Immunohistochemical distinction between mesothelial and adenocarcinoma cells in serous effusions: A combination panel-based approach with a brief review of the literature. Indian Journal of Pathology & Microbiology. 2009;**52**(2):175

[53] Dejmek A, Hjerpe A. Reactivity of six antibodies in effusions of mesothelioma, adenocarcinoma and mesotheliosis: Stepwise logistic regression analysis. Cytopathology. 2000;**11**(1):8-17

[54] Su X-Y, Li G-D, Liu W-P, Xie B, Jiang Y-H. Cytological differential diagnosis among adenocarcinoma, epithelial mesothelioma, and reactive mesothelial cells in serous effusions by immunocytochemistry. Diagnostic Cytopathology. 2011;**39**(12):900-908

[55] Bailey ME, Brown RW, Mody DR, Cagle P, Ramzy I. Ber-EP4 for differentiating adenocarcinoma from reactive and neoplastic mesothelial cells in serous effusions. Acta Cytologica. 1996;**40**(6):1212-1216

[56] Sheahan K, O'brien MJ, Burke B, Dervan PA, O'brien JC, Gottlieb LS, et al. Differential Reactivities of carcinoembryonic antigen (CEA) and CEA-related monoclonal and polyclonal antibodies in common epithelial malignancies. American Journal of Clinical Pathology. 1990;**94**(2):157-164

[57] Jo VY, Cibas ES, Pinkus GS. Claudin-4 immunohistochemistry

is highly effective in distinguishing adenocarcinoma from malignant mesothelioma in effusion cytology. Cancer Cytopathology. 2014;**122**(4):299-306

[58] Vojtek M, Walsh MD, Papadimos DJ, Shield PW. Claudin-4 immunohistochemistry is a useful pan-carcinoma marker for serous effusion specimens. Cytopathology. 2019 Nov;**30**(6):614-619

[59] Ordóñez NG. Value of Claudin-4 immunostaining in the diagnosis of mesothelioma. American Journal of Clinical Pathology. 2013;**139**(5):611-619

[60] Dashti S, Heidarpour M, Afshar-Moghaddam N. Diagnostic value of claudin-4 marker in pleural and peritoneal effusion cytology: Does it differentiate between metastatic adenocarcinoma and reactive mesothelial cells? Advanced Biomedical Research. 2014;**3**(1):161

[61] Lonardi S, Manera C, Marucci R, Santoro A, Lorenzi L, Facchetti F. Usefulness of Claudin 4 in the cytological diagnosis of serosal effusions. Diagnostic Cytopathology. 2011;**39**(5):313-317

[62] Sauter JL, Bueno R, Dacic S, Gill RR, Husain AN, Kadota K, et al. Diffuse Plaural mesothelioma. In: Thoracic Tumours WHO, editor. Classification of Tumours. 5th ed. Lyon: WHO Classification of Tumours Editorial Board; 2021. pp. 204-219

[63] Stevers M, Rabban JT, Garg K, Van Ziffle J, Onodera C, Grenert JP, et al. Well-differentiated papillary mesothelioma of the peritoneum is genetically defined by mutually exclusive mutations in TRAF7 and CDC42. Modern Pathology. 2019;**32**(1):88-99

[64] Clarke JM, Helft P. Long-term survival of a woman with well differentiated papillary mesothelioma of the peritoneum: A case report and review of the literature. Journal of Medical Case Reports. 2010;**4**(1):346

[65] Rathi V, Hyde S, Newman M. Well-differentiated papillary mesothelioma in association with endometrial carcinoma: A case report. Acta Cytologica. 2010;**54**(5 Suppl):793-797

[66] Butnor KJ, Roden AC, Tazelaar HDWJ. Well-differentiated papillary mesothelial tumor of the pleura. In: Thoracic Tumours WHO Classification of Tumours. 5th ed. Lyon: WHO Classification of Tumours Editorial Board; 2021. pp. 198-199

[67] Beasley MB, Galateau-Salle F, Dacic S. Pleural mesothelioma classification update. Virchows Archiv. 2021;**478**(1):59-72

[68] Oramas DM, Zaleski M, Moran CA. Sarcomatoid mesothelioma: A Clinicopathological and Immunohistochemical study of 64 cases. International Journal of Surgical Pathology. 2021;**29**(8):820-825

Chapter 4

Fibulin-3 as a Biomarker of Pleuric Involvement by Exposure to Fibers

Venerando Antonio Rapisarda and Caterina Ledda

Abstract

This chapter deals extensively with the role of Fibulin-3 (Fb-3) as early marker of malignant development, triggered by direct and long exposure to asbestos or asbestiform fibers. Asbestos has widely been used in many civic and industrial environments. Despite numerous countries, e.g., the European Union and the United States, have forbidden its production as well as utilization, still nowadays millions of tons of asbestos are manufactured worldwide. When inhaled, it causes the onset of malignant mesothelioma (MM) and several other types of cancer, including lung cancer. Health surveillance of subjects formerly exposed to asbestos is based on an early detection of major asbestos-related pathologies. However, the protocols adopted so far do not meet the sensitivity and specificity requirements needed to ensure an early diagnosis. Among the various eligible MM biomarkers, scientists have recently proposed Fb-3, which is a glycoprotein belonging to extracellular matrix proteins, coded through EFEMP-1 gene 2p 16 chromosome). Fb-3 is expressed by mesenchymal cells and plays a role in angiogenic processes as well-regulating cell-to-cell and cell-to-extra cellular matrix communication. However, it is weakly expressed also in healthy tissues. Previous studies conducted on MM historically asbestos-exposed patients have shown, on several biological matrixes such as serum and plasma, high Fb-3 concentrations. In the same way, high levels of circulating Fb-3 were observed in subjects exposed to a natural asbestiform fiber called fluoro-edenite (FE). Direct association between an increased Fb-3 expression and exposure to FE fibers has also been found in *in-vitro* and *ex-vivo* studies.

Keywords: fibulin-3, mesothelioma, asbestos, asbestos like fibers, biomarker

1. Introduction

Malignant mesothelioma (MM) is a malignant tumor originating from the mesothelial layer of the pleura, peritoneum, pericardium, and vaginal tunic and traditionally related to the exposure to asbestos fibers [1]. Asbestos includes different types of minerals: serpentine (chrysotile), and fibrous amphiboles cummingtonite-grunerite (amosite asbestos), actinolite, anthophyllite, riebeckite (crocidolite asbestos), anthracite, and tremolite. Such fibers represent an environmental health problem as chronic exposure to these minerals has been associated with respiratory diseases, including cancer. Additionally, exposure to several other types of mineral particles found in the natural environment and termed "naturally occurring asbestos" (NOA) such as fibers of the minerals erionite, winchite, magnesio-riebeckite, Libby asbestos, richterite, antigorite, and fluoro-edenite (FE) have also been associated with MM [1, 2].

At present, MM is still considered a lethal cancer characterized by a considerable period of latency (≥30–60 years) and late diagnosis that determines bad prognosis and quality of life and unresponsiveness to presently available treatments [3]. To date, there are no diagnostic tools with high sensitivity and specificity that can be used to perform an early diagnosis of MM in asymptomatic people. Many biomarkers have been proposed for the screening and diagnosis of MM in exposed subjects [3–13]. Pathogenic mechanisms of lung illness were linked to the activation of different biomarkers including fibulin-3 (Fb-3) [3].

2. Fibulin-3 (Fb-3) gene expression

Fb-3 also known as Epidermal Growth Factor (EGF) Containing Fibulin Extracellular Matrix Protein-1 (EFEMP1) is an extracellular glycoprotein generally expressed in most tissues already in their embryonic phase. It is one of the seven proteins that belong to fibulinic family. Fibulins are characterized by EGF-like domain-couple *calcium-binding-cb* layout (epidermal growth factor) and a C-terminal *fibulin type* module. Fb-3 is codified by the EFEMP1 gene (also known as S1–5) present in chromosome 2p16. EFEMP1 contains 11 exons and codifies for a protein of 493 aminoacids with a 55 kDa molecular mass [14].

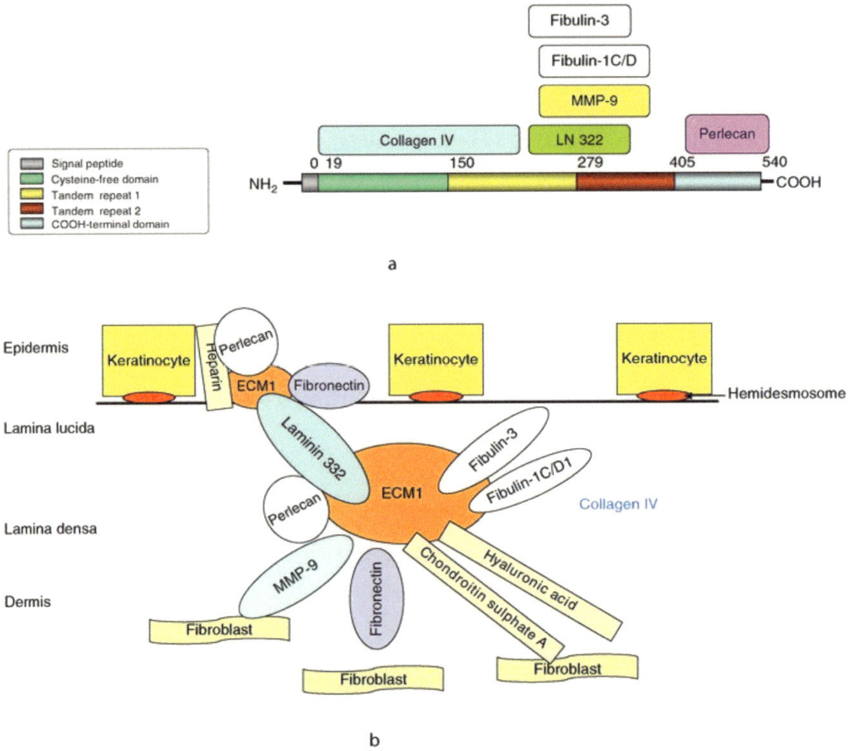

Figure 1.
Expression of Fb-3 in relation to the structures of the cellular matrix (by textbook of aging skin springer).

The protein sequence contains a signaling peptide, five cbEGF domain couples preceded by a modified cbEGF domain and a *fibulin-type* C-terminal module. The modified cbEGF domain features an insert of 88 aminoacids. Under physiological conditions, Fb-3 is found in monomeric form. The recombining Fb-3 shows a small shaft-like structure with a globule at one of its ends, which probably consists of the cbEGF modified domain [15].

Fb-3, like many other molecules that form the base membrane, has preserved itself best among the several species, keeping 92–94% of aminoacids identical in human, rats, and mice. During growth process, Fb-3 is expressed at mesenchyme level, especially in bone and cartilage structures.

In studies on Fb-3, the EFEMP1 gene was originally cloned by senescent fibroblasts taken from a subject with Werner Syndrome, a disease characterized by early aging, where an EFEMP1 mRNA overexpression can be observed. However, no mutation or fault in the EFEMP1 gene has been associated with Werner Syndrome or any other aging factors [16].

In adults, Fb-3 is largely distributed in various tissues, including the eyes. Particularly, a high expression of this glycoprotein can be observed in epithelial and endothelial cells, in their base membrane (see **Figure 1**) [1].

The latter play an essential role not only in structural or filtering functions, such as kidney glomerules, but also because they come into play in determining cell polarity and regulating cellular metabolic, proliferation, differentiation, and migration processes.

3. Fb-3 action mechanism

Fb-3 interacts with other base membrane proteins, such as extracellular matrix 1 protein (ECM1), the tissue inhibitor of metalloproteinase-3 (TIMP-3), endostatine (20 kDa C-terminal fragment of collagene XVIII), B hepatitis virus antigene X, tropoelastine (elastine monomeric subunit), etc. These interactions are likely to contribute to maintaining the base membrane integrity and anchoring other ECM structures, e.g., elastic fibers [17].

Fb-3 stimulates TIMP-1 and TIMP-3 expressions, but it inhibits expression and activities of (MMP)-2, MMP-3 and MMP-9 matrix metalloproteinases. It is associated with thinner elastic fibers, whereas it is not found in bigger elastic structures such as the aortic elastic lamina. Experimental studies have highlighted that EFEMp1 *knockout* rats show an early aging process and develop multiple tissue hernias, among which inguinal hernias, pelvic prolapse, and xiphoid process protrusions. In these guinea pigs, small-size elastic fibers of the connective tissue, including those of small blood vessel adventitia and vaginal tunics, are reduced both in size and resistance. A disgregation or a reduction of the elastic fibers in such tissues is probably responsible for phenotypes suffering from early aging and multiple hernias observed in *knockout* rats for EFEMP1.

Besides its role in maintaining ECM, Fb-3 also seems to have signaling functions. Indeed, Fb-3, by interacting with DA41, a protein, which binds the onco-suppressor DAN gene, can trigger DNA synthesis. The expression of EFEMP1 is thought to have a role in cell proliferation and tissue growth processes [18].

Inactivation of EFEMP1, through promoter methylation methylation of the stimulator, is associated with lung and breast cancers. EFEMP1 undergoes a *down-regulation* in 60% of breast cancer cases and the promoter methylation methylation of the stimulator just seems to be the main reason for this reduced expression. Analysis of primary primitive, clinically well-characterized breast cancers has revealed a significant correlation between a reduced EFEMP1 expression and a reduction of the time span free from illness and of survival, generally. In the light of this evidence, one can assume that EFEMP1 might be used as molecular marker in lung and breast cancers.

An alteration of Fb-3, as an element of the base membrane, would seem to play an important role in tumor metastatic phenomena. Fb-3 would also seem to have a triggering action in cellular proliferation and migration processes. However, both the pathophysiological role of Fb-3 in base membranes and how the alteration and/or function failure of this protein may/may not have a part in causing pathologies are still to be ascertained.

4. Lab procedures to determine Fb-3

4.1 Fb-evaluation from tissues

Immunohistochemistry (IHC) is a laboratory technique, which enables to highlight the creation of antigen–antibody complexes inside a tissue.

Such diagnosis technique exploits the ability of some antibodies to recognize cellular proteins (like Fb-3), called antigens, which in tumoral cells may have expression characteristics (more or less apparent) other than those of ordinary cells. The sample, after fomalin paraffin fixation and inclusion, is prepared for the immunohistochemical exam first by de-paraffining the sections, then remoisturizing them, and finally submitting them to antigenic unmasking. The sample is then incubated with the primary antibody and then with by a biotine-streptovidina-kit detection system. To visualize the immunoreaction, Diaminobenzidine (DAB) is used as chromogen, which highlights the immunolabeling in brown. Densimetric and morphometric analyses of Fb-3 are obtained through optical microscope and image analysis software reading, in order to assess density in pixels (% of unit density) and the percentage of pixel immuno-labeled areas of the above quoted protein (see **Figure 2**) [2].

4.2 Assessment of Fb-3 from serum, plasma and other biological liquids

ELISA stands for Enzyme Linked Immuno Sorbent Assay. It is an immunological analysis technique used to assess any evidence of a particular antigen in a sample.

ELISA combines the specificity of the antigen antibody reaction (immunological reaction) with the sensibility of a simple enzyme spectrophotometric dosage (see **Figure 3**).

Such technique is based on the assumption that, with adequate procedures, it is possible to conjugate the antibodies of a serum with some enzymes (peroxidase, alcalin phosphatase, beta-galactosidase) without altering their property to combine with the correspondent antigens. The enzyme used can catalyze a reaction on a suitable substratum with the formation of a colored terminal product, which allows highlighting the quantity of the antigen. In commercial formats, reactions are usually carried out inside polyvinyl or polystyrene wells (12 strip microplates with 8 wells each for a total of 96 wells) on which specific antibodies are attached for the antigen of interest or the antigen itself. The samples to analyze (plasma, serum, pleural liquid, broncho-aspirate, bronchoalveolar lavage, etc.) as well as reagents with interspersed

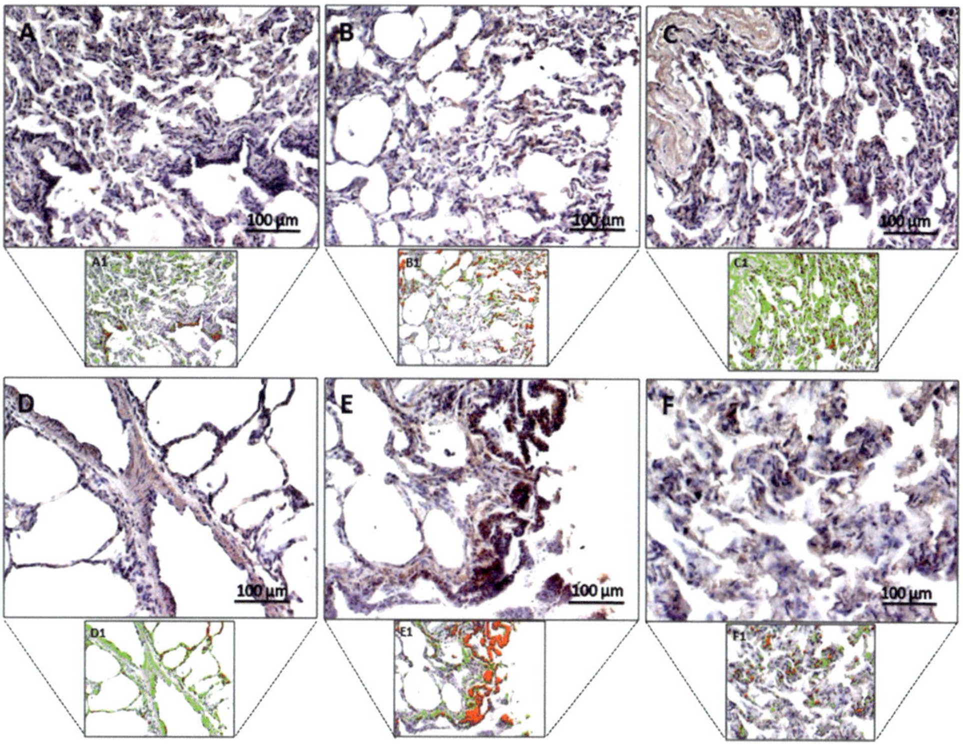

Figure 2.
Figure. IHC determination of Fb-3 in lung tissues exposed to fluoro-edenite (FE). A–F: Sections of exposed lung tissue in which Fb-3 immunoexpression was detected in intraparenchymal stroma around bronchioles, bronchiolar epithelium, interstitium between alveoli, alveolar epithelium, and macrophages. A1-F1: Image analysis by software in which an evident both high (red color) and low (green color) immunostaining was detected in exposed lung. A-F, original magnification 20x; scale bar: 100 μm.

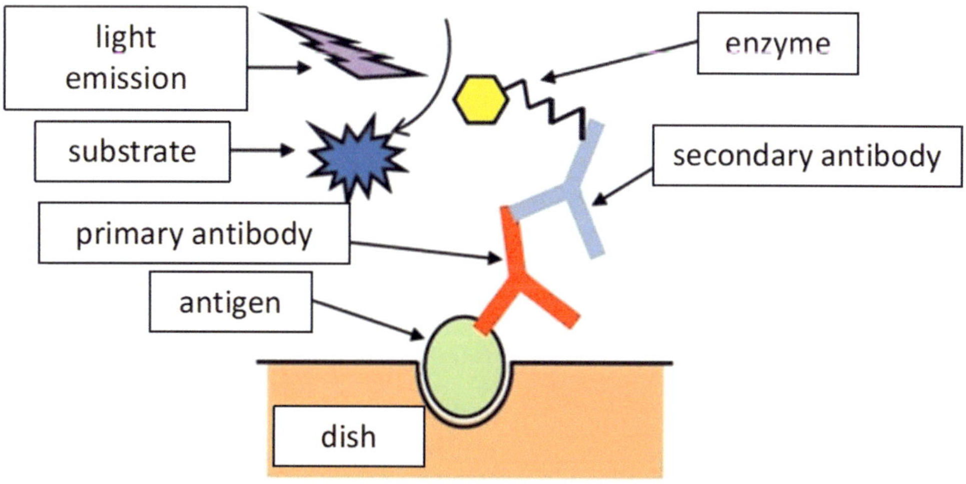

Figure 3.
Schematic drawing showing the antigen–antibody reaction (immunological reaction).

lavages needed to remove any excess are incubated inside these wells. Lastly, the substratum is added, which generates the colored product.

Positivity is assessed analyzing occurrence or not of the color, following the reaction catalyzed by the enzyme on the substratum. Immunoenzymatic technique can be used for researching both antigens and antibodies and lends itself to several variations for numerous applications likewise.

5. Fb-3 as biomarker in asbestos-related pathologies

One of the earliest studies involving the role of Fb-3 in cancer was carried out in 2009 in the United States on gliomas [19]. Following some preliminary investigations, the authors had hypothesized that gliomas' local invasiveness could be caused by an interaction between mesenchymal proteins and some specific neural matrix proteins. In fact, unlike other central neuro system neoplasms (CNS), characterized by an expansive growth with shifting and compression of the surrounding parenchyma, gliomas show an infiltration type of growth. The extracellular matrix in the CNS normally contains high quantities of ialuronic acid and negatively charged proteoglycans, but low quantities of fibrillar proteins, which may support cellular adherence and mobility. In an attempt to identify the humoral signs, which could contribute to gliomas' peculiar invasiveness (probably due to an altered relationship between cells and extracellular matrix), researchers have stimulated tumoral cells *in-vitro,* combining mesenchymal elements (fibronectine) with others, specific of the neural matrix (brevican) and, by using a micro-array, examined which genes came out overexpressed. Results showed a remarkable rise of Fb-3 expression in the glioma.

Successive studies about the role of Fb-3 showed mixed results: some observed an antagonist effect toward tumoral angiogenesis (reducing so its aggressiveness); others, as in the case of pancreatic adenocarcinomas and gliomas, observed Fb-3 expression rise associated with an increased vascular growth factor (VEGF) and tumoral growth. **Table 1** reports some studies on Fb-3 and of different kind of cancers.

A research of 2011 on colorectal cancer detected an Fb-3 *downregulation* in the cancerous tissues compared with the adjacent healthy ones. Furthermore, the Fb-3 *downregulation* negatively correlated with the prognosis, tumor stage, lympho-node metastatis, and reduced time gaps free from the illness.

In a following study, Fb-3 plasma levels were tested in colon-cancer subjects, comparing them with a control group made up of healthy subjects. The Fb-3 resulted significantly reduced in tumor-stricken subjects, in a directly proportional manner with lymphonode metastases and, at length, the tumoral mass and in general with the neoplasm stage.

In intestinal tumors, Fb-3 *downregulation* seems then to show a worsened prognosis due to a reduced anti-angiogenic action.

In the light of what has been said, Fb-3 is thought to play, depending on the tumor type, a pro-angiogenic role (gliomas, cervix carcinoma) or an anti-angiogenic one (colon carcinoma). This apparent paradox may derive from a different behavior of this glycoprotein in relation to factors such as tissue histological characteristics and tumor micro-environment. The Fb-3 bond with TIMP-3 might interfere with that between VEGF to its type 2 receptor (VEGFR-2), causing the inhibition of tumoral angiogenesis. Besides, it has been observed that Fb-3 is able to competitively link the EGF receptor (EGFR) compared with EGF, so activating intra-cellular pathways (MAPK, Akt) in pancreatic adenocarcinoma. Finally, a few studies have concluded that the

Authors	Cancer type	Fb-3 regulation	Applied technology
Pass et al. [3]	MM	Up	IHC and ELISA
Jiang et al. [4]	MM	Up	IHC
Hassan et al. [5]	MM	Up	ELISA
Caltabiano et al. [6]	MM	Up	IHC
Jiang et al. [7]	MM	Up	ELISA
Battolla et al. [8]	MM	Up	ELISA
Napolitano et al. [9]	MM	Up	ELISA
Kirschner et al. [10]	MM	Up	ELISA
Kaya et al. [11]	MM	Up	ELISA
Creaney et al. [12]	MM	Up	ELISA
Corradi et al. [13]	MM	Up	ELISA
Pass et al. [3]	Ovarian	Down	IHC and ELISA
Pass et al. [3]	Glioblastoma	Down	IHC and ELISA
Nandhu et al. [17]	Glioblastoma	Up	IHC and rt-PCR
Hu et al. [19]	Glioblastoma	Up	IHC and rt-PCR
Pass et al. [3]	Prostatic	Down	IHC and ELISA
Hassan et al. [5]	Lung	Down	ELISA
Chen et al. [20]	Lung	Down	IHC and rt-PCR
Corradi et al. [13]	Lung	Down	ELISA
Wang et al. [21]	Cutaneous squamous	Down	IHC
Hwang et al. [22]	Nasopharyngeal	Down	IHC
Luo et al. [16]	Hepatocellular	Down	IHC and rt-PCR
Kim et al. [23]	Pancreatic	Down	ELISA
Li et al. [24]	Cervix	Up	IHC and ICC
Wang et al. [25]	Osteosarcoma	Up	IHC and ICC
Han et al. [26]	Bladder	Up	IHC and rt-PCR
Simsek et al. [27]	Colorectal	Down	ELISA
Tong et al. [28]	Colorectal	Down	IHC
Tian et al. [29]	Breast	Down	IHC
Noonan et al. [30]	Breast	Up	ELISA

rt-PCR = reverse transcriptase polymerase chain reaction; ICC = immunocytochemistry.

Table 1.
Studies exploring Fb-3 in relation to cancer type.

EFEMP1 gene activation, due to the hypermethylation of its promoter, also occurs in several cancer types (lung, prostatic, colorectal, nasopharyngeal, and hepatocellular).

These data seem to point out that a reduced expression of this gene may be involved in carcinogenic and/or tumor growth processes. It seems however evident how the exact role of Fb-3 in tumoral growth still remains to be clarified and needs further research.

Recent studies on the pathophysiological role of Fb-3 in malignant mesothelioma (MM) are also taking into account this glycoprotein as a possible marker for early diagnosis and/or pathology follow-up.

This research falls within a larger assessment context of potential biomarkers in MM early diagnosis.

MM is a fatal tumor, with a long latency and aspecific symptoms, which often end up in a late diagnosis. MM is causally correlated with exposure to asbestos or asbestiform fibers. MM cases worldwide are definitely increasing. In Italy, an incidence peak is expected within 2025 [31, 32].

Actually 25% of MM is caused by professional exposure, 25% through indirect exposure of family members, and 50% from exposure to fibers in the surrounding environment [33].

MM patients survive averagely 6–18 months from diagnosis. However, it has been noticed that, if an early diagnosis is made, survival may even go beyond 5 years. Unfortunately, today there are still no effective prevention systems and screening procedures for this pathology [31–34].

Periodical X-ray exams have always been hard to do, due to: long latency of the disease (14–45 years); limited resolution of present techniques, especially for lesions at an early stage; exposure to ionizing radiations (justification principle). It is then clear how finding humoral biomarkers with high sensitivity and specificity might significantly enhance the prognosis of this disease.

Scientific debate on the eligible molecules has been going on for long, with no definite results. Indeed, none of the biomarkers studied seems to meet the requirements needed [35, 36].

The first study to propose using Fb-3 as a possible MM biomarker was conducted by Pass et al. [3]. The intent of the study was to analyze Fb-3 reliability compared with mesothelin, a protein already thoroughly studied as a biomarker, which had however shown no adequate sensitivity (47%) in recognizing MM cases. Plasma and effusion samples from patients with pleural MM, plasma samples from persons who had been exposed to asbestos but did not have MM, and plasma and effusion samples from patients with pleural effusions not due to MM were analyzed.

In this study performed on MM patients, sampling was carried out in the United States, at the Wayne State University, from 1998 to 2005, and at New York University Langone Medical Center, from 2005 to 2011, the "Detroit Cohort" and the "New York Cohort," respectively.

The study also assessed patients with other neoplasms, in order to improve Fb-3 specificity. Altogether, 20 ovarian cancer, 20 glioblastoma, and 31 prostatic carcinoma patients were evaluated. Furthermore, 43 healthy subjects were used as control group (selection criteria included absence of previous exposure to asbestos and other neoplastic pathologies).

In conclusion, plasma Fb-3 levels can distinguish healthy persons with exposure to asbestos from patients with MM. In conjunction with effusion Fb-3 levels, plasma Fb-3 levels can further differentiate MM effusions from other malignant and benign effusions [3].

On the whole, there were 11 studies dealing with concentrations of Fb-3 in human beings, and they were performed on: MM tumoral tissue; pleural exudate; serum and plasma (see **Table 2**).

The surveys on MM patients' tumoral tissues were conducted by Pass et al. [3] and Caltabiano et al. [6].

Authors	Explored matrix	Patient's pathology/exposure (n.)
Agha et al. [37]	Pleural exudate and plasma	MM (25), pleural exudate by no-MM neoplastic pathologies (11); benign pleura lesions (9).
Battolla et al. [8]	Pleural exudate	MM (33); pleural exudate by no-MM neoplastic pathologies (23); benign pleura lesions (64).
Creaney et al. [12]	Pleural exudate and plasma	MM (82); pleural exudate by no-MM neoplastic pathologies (36); benign pleura lesions (35).
Corradi et al. [13]	Plasma	MM (50); lung cancer (77); benign lung lesions (16); healthy control (66).
Demir et al. [36]	Serum	MM (42); healthy control not exposure to asbestos (48); healthy control exposure to asbestos (48);
Hassan et al. [5]	Serum	MM (45); lung cancer (63); benign lung lesions (63); benign pleura lesions (48); healthy control (60).
Jiang et al. [7]	Plasma	MM (15); benign lung lesions (29); benign pleura lesions (74); exposed to asbestos with no lesions (218); healthy control (94).
Kaya et al. [11]	Serum	MM (43); healthy control (40).
Kirschner et al. [10]	Plasma	MM (114); no MM cancers (37); benign pleura lesions (45); cardiac pathologies (34).
Napolitano et al. [9]	Plasma	MM (22); pleural exudate by no-MM neoplastic pathologies (25); benign pleura lesions (13); healthy control (20).
Pass et al. [3]	Pleural exudate and plasma	MM (92); exposed to asbestos with no lesions (136); benign pleura lesions (93); healthy control (43).

Table 2.
Studies exploring Fb-3 in pleural fluids and peripheral blood.

In Pass et al. [3], the immunohistochemical analysis enabled to give a score to the nuclear as well as to the citoplasmatic positivity, taking into account both the number of positive cells and the positivity intensity. The authors detected Fb-3 nuclear and citoplasmatic expression in 100% of MM samples (26/26); the scores for intensity were similar both for the epithelial subtype, and the sarcomatoid and the sarcomatoid/epithelial mixed variant ones.

Comparison among the epithelial-histological, the epithelial-biphasic-histological and the sarcomatoid subtypes showed similar scores as far as the coloring intensity was concerned (mean score 7.7 ± 0.6 and 6.9 ± 0.8, respectively $P = 0.87$); and so did it with purely sarcomatoid- histological subtypes (6.6 ± 1.1; $P = 0.62$). The total coloring score (nuclear and citoplasmatic) turned out constantly higher in MM samples than in those detected in other pleural neoplastic forms (7.4 ± 0.5 vs. 2.4 ± 0.8; $P < 0.001$).

In Caltabiano et al. [6], Fb-3 immunohistochemical expression was assessed on tumoral tissues of six MM patients, previously exposed to fluoroedenite (FE); a natural, asbestiform fiber discovered in lava rock stone used as construction material in Biancavilla's municipality, on the slopes of Mount Etna.

Outcomes showed immunoexpression similar in the epithelial histological subtypes (three cases) and in the epithelial biphasic histological and sarcomatoid subtype (three cases) (see **Figure 4**).

The analysis of Fb-3 concentration in the pleural exudate was carried out in four studies: Pass et al. [3]; Creaney et al., [12]; Agha et al. [37]; Battolla et al. [8].

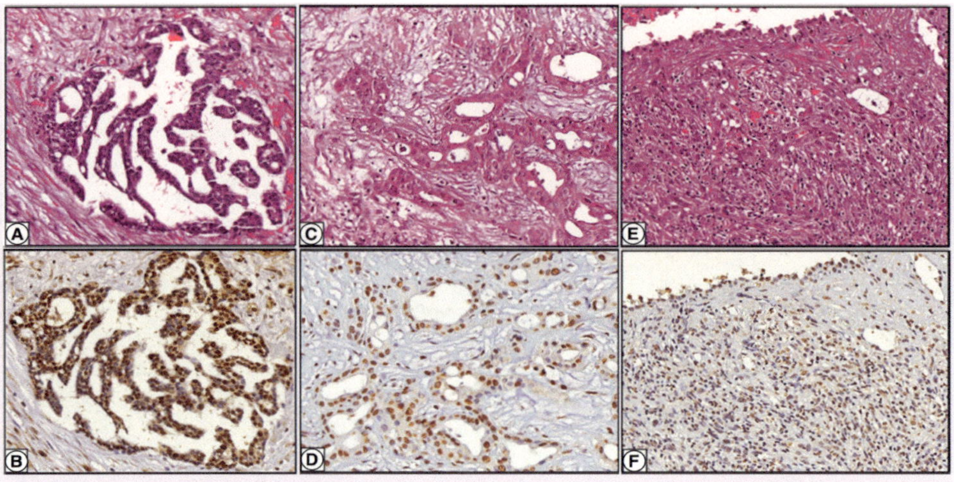

Figure 4.
IHC expression of Fb-3. (A) Hematoxylin and eosin (H&E) stained section of an epithelioid mesothelioma composed of glandular structures exhibiting diffuse and strong staining for Fb-3 (B). Immunohistochemical staining for Fb-3 in the same case depicted in (A): Neoplastic cells within glandular structures exhibit diffuse and strong nuclear and cytoplasmic staining for Fb-3. (C) H&E stained section of another case of epithelioid mesothelioma composed of closely packed glands showing diffuse and moderate staining for Fb-3 (D). Immunohistochemical staining for Fb-3 in the same case depicted in (B): Neoplastic cells show a diffuse staining for Fb-3 of moderate intensity. (E) H&E section of a biphasic mesothelioma composed predominantly of neoplastic spindle-shaped cells; (F) this case exhibited a diffuse staining for Fb-3; however, the staining intensity was recorded as weak.

Pass et al. [3] observed significantly higher concentrations of Fb-3 in MM subjects' pleural exudate than those detected in benign exudates or derived from other neoplasms. Therefore, the Fb-3 concentration allowed to tell MM subjects from all the others (area below the curve-AUC = 0.93), both in benign (AUC = 0.93) and in malignant pathologies (AUC = 0.94). Moreover, Fb-3 levels did not significantly differ between those patients (n = 22) who had received presurgery chemotherapy and those (52) who had not (617.4 ± 72.5 vs. 703.6 ± 42.6 ng/ml).

Fb-3 significantly correlated with the progress of the disease and made it possible to distinguish those patients (n = 54) who underwent citoreductive surgery in stage I-II (n = 21), from those (n = 33) with III-IV stage disease (576 ± 67 ng/ml vs. 765 ± 55 ng/ml, P = 0.04).

An Fb-3 = 733.4 ng/ml cutoff, measured at the time of surgery in all subjects (n = 69), correlated in an inverse proportional way with patients' survival.

Creaney et al. [12] detected Fb-3 values and mesotheline in the pleural exudate of 153 patients: 82 had MM, 36 had pleural exudate caused by other neoplastic pathologies; 35 had benign exudates.

The MM patients' samples were collected within a month from diagnosis, prior to any kind of treatment. Fb-3 levels ranged between 17 and 5748 ng/ml. No significant difference was detected in Fb-3 levels among the three groups under exam; in detail, 63% of benign exudate samples exceeded the 346 ng/ml cutoff. Statistical analysis showed no difference in Fb-3 levels according to the pleural liquid protein composition (exudate or drained) and/or with blood.

Exudates coming from MM patients with biphasic or sarcomatoid histology showed significantly higher levels of Fb-3 (1331, range 538–2486 ng/ml) than the epithelial ones (426, range 171–1709 ng/ml; P = 0.018), also in those patients who had

had a citological-based diagnosis (298, range 155–881 ng/ml; P = 0.002). No significant difference was observed in Fb-3 levels according to the stage of the disease. Altogether, the Fb-3 study results in the pleural exudate showed a 59% sensitivity and a 52% specificity, considering 346 ng/ml. as threshold. The 0.588 AUC enabled to tell MM patients from all the others.

As regards mesothelin levels, they were remarkably higher in MM patients than in those with benign exudates (P < 0.001) and in others with exudates caused by other neoplasms (P < 0,001).

Creaney and colleagues concluded that mesothelin gave out a 58% sensitivity and a 96% specificity, as well as a better diagnostic accuracy, compared with Fb-3 in pleural exudates of MM patients.

A study carried out by Agha et al. [37] analyzed 45 patients with pleural exudate, of whom: 25 MM cases, 11 secondary pleural metastases (3 cases of not-small-cell lung cancer, 2 breast cancers, 3 colon cancers, 1 case of kidney cancer, and 2 cases of limphoma), and 9 patients with benign origin pleural exudates (5 tubercolosis, 1 pneumonia, and 3 pleurisies). MM patients showed significantly higher Fb-3 levels (331 ± 32.64 ng/ml) than those with pleural exudate derived from secondary metastases (153.01 ± 60.32 ng/ml). The difference between these parameters turned out to be statistically significant (P < 0.001).

The results highlighted that with a 150 ng/ml cut-off (AUC = 0.878; 72.3% sensitivity, 80% specificity), it was possible to tell MM patients from those with pleural metastatic pathology.

Besides, exploiting a 127.5 ng/ml cut-off (AUC = 0.909; sensitivity 88%, specificity 77.8%) it was possible to distinguish MM from the pleural benign exudate.

In a recent study, Battolla et al. compared Fb-3 and mesothelin levels in MM patients' pleural liquid with that obtained from patients with pleural pathologies, both benign and malignant, other than MM. 120 subjects underwent thoracenthesis between 2008 and 2011. Among these, 33 had MM, 64 had benign pleura lesions and 23 secondary pleural metastases. Fb-3 and mesothelin concentrations were assessed in ELISA. Results showed Fb-3 levels substantially similar in all subjects (P = 0.174), whereas mesothelin levels were significantly higher in MM subjects than others (P = 0.001).

The analysis of Fb-3 concentration in peripheral blood was conducted in seven surveys on plasma and three on serum.

In Pass et al.'s study (2012), Fb-3 plasma values were assessed. The study sample included: 92 MM patients; 136 exposed to asbestos with no cancer; 93 patients with nonrelated MM pleural exudate; 43 healthy subjects as control group. The study was carried out in two separate cohorts: "Detroit cohort" and "New York cohort."

Outcomes highlighted that Fb-3 average plasma levels enabled to significantly distinguish asbestos-exposed subjects from those with nonrelated MM exudate and from MM ones, in both cohorts. Fb-3 concentrations in MM "Detroit cohort" patients were similar to those of the "New York cohort" (105.0 ± 7.1 vs. 112.9 ± 7.6 ng/ml; P = 0.63). Fb-3 plasma levels did not significantly differ between the 44 MM patients, who had had presurgery chemotherapy and the 48 who had not (117.9 ± 8.1 vs. 101.1 ± 6.9 ng/ml; P = 0.12).

Fb-3 plasma level allowed to tell MM patients from those affected from other cancers or even those with pleural exudate (not MM-related), both benign and malignant. Finally, comparing the 28 patients at stage I-II of MM with the asbestos-exposed ones, with AUC = 0.99 and cutoff = 46.0 ng/ml, a 100% sensitivity [95% IC,

87.7–100] and a 94.1% specificity [95% IC, from 88.7 to 97.4] were reached. Fb-3 levels of MM patients went down after surgery in 100% of cases (18 out of 18).

Contrary to expectations, the authors found poor correlation between Fb-3 levels found in plasma samples and those detected in the pleural exudate of each MM patient (n = 17) (P = 0.98), as well as in the plasma and pleural exudate of 15 patients who had not MM-related exudate (P = 0.27).

Among the conclusions, the authors suggested using plasma samples instead of serum ones so as to assess Fb-3 blood levels, since the presence of two potential trombine cleavage sites could compromise the validity of the exam. Despite the encouraging results obtained by Pass's survey, further experiments gave out mixed outcomes.

A cohort of 153 patients (of whom 82 having MM) was investigated by Creaney et al., reporting a 22% sensitivity and a 95% specificity for plasma Fb-3 (cutoff = 52 ng/ml, AUC = 0.671). These values were definitely lower than those obtained, with the same patients for mesothelin (sensitivity 56%; specificity 95%—AUC = 0.816), which on the contrary seems to have a decisively better diagnostic accuracy on plasma samples. Although in this study mesothelin resulted superior to Fb-3 as to its diagnostic worth, the authors considered the latter superior from a prognostic point of view. Indeed, Fb-3 high levels correlated negatively with the patient's prognosis. A possible explanation of this might depend on an Fb-3 higher expression by biphasic and sarcomatoid histotypes, which are generally characterized by a worse prognosis. Instead, mesothelin is mainly expressed by the epithelial histotype, with a better prognosis.

An Egyptian study [37] conducted on a small cohort of 45 subjects reported a 100% sensitivity and a 78% specificity in differentiating MM cases (n = 25) from nonmalignant pleural pathologies (n = 9), and an 88% sensitivity and 82% specificity in distinguishing MM from other forms of pleural cancer (n = 11). It is necessary, though, to point out that the authors, when evaluating Fb-3, used a nonspecified test and internally agreed cutoffs.

Corradi et al. assessed the concentration of Fb-3 and other protein biomarkers in the serum of four groups of patients: subjects previously exposed to asbestos and suffering from asbestosis; patients with MM; patients with not-small-cell lung carcinoma (NSCLC) and a control group, which showed no evidence of neoplastic pathologies. The results highlighted higher levels of Fb-3 in MM patients than the NSCLC group (P < 0.01) and the control (P < 0.05). However, Fb-3 values in MM patients did not significantly differ from those of subjects with asbestosis. The small number of patients in the study is the main weakness of these results.

A prospective survey carried out by Kaya et al. [11] examined 43 MM patients (primary involvement: 39 pleural, 4 peritoneal mesothelioma) and 40 controls. Results showed Fb-3 serum levels equal to 90.3 ± 42.1 and 17.8 ± 12.7 ng/ml, respectively (P < 0.001). A 36.6 ng/ml cutoff indicated a 93% sensitivity and a 90% specificity.

Napolitano et al. [9] analyzed levels of *high mobility group box protein* 1 (HMGB1) and Fb-3 in blood samples of 22 MM subjects, 20 others with documented exposure to asbestos, 13 with benign pleural exudate, 25 with malignant exudate (other than MM) and 20 controls. The authors concluded that the combination of HMGB1 and Fb-3 provided higher sensitivity and specificity in differentiating MM patients from others with benign or malignant pleural pathologies.

MM etiology usually involves professional and/or environmental exposure to asbestos. In an attempt to spot any possible differences among the MM types derived after environmental exposure, compared to the more frequently documented professional one, Demir et al. recruited a cohort of MM patients (n = 42) derived after

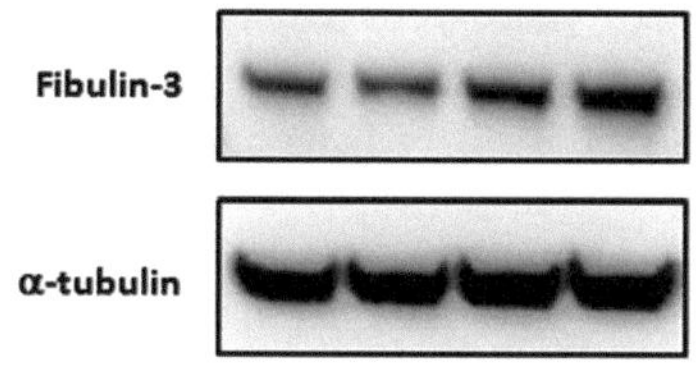

Figure 5.
Western blot analysis of Fb-3 protein level evaluated in primary human lung fibroblasts exposed to 10, 50 and 100 μg/ml of FE fibers for 72 h.

environmental exposure to asbestos and compared them with two control groups: the former composed of healthy individuals (n = 48) who had no previous, documented exposure to asbestos, with a normal chest X-ray exam; the latter, (n = 48) composed of subjects with documented environmental exposure to asbestos for at least 15 years, who showed no X-ray documented pleural plaques. The authors detected significantly higher values of Fb-3 in MM patients' serum than in those who were just exposed to asbestos and the nonexposed control group.

Several investigations conducted by the working group (Caltabiano, Ledda and Loreto) directed by Rapisarda et al. [1, 6, 38, 39] analyzed the role of Fb-3 as biomarker in workers exposed to FE. Fb-3 plasma concentrations were measured in the blood of the FE-exposed workers and in a control group (non-exposed). In 52% of exposed subjects pleural plaques were detected. Fb-3 plasma concentrations resulted 12.96 e 5.29 ng/ml, respectively, in the exposed subjects compared to the control ($P < 0.001$).

The results highlighted a high predictive value of Fb-3 plasma levels in relation to the presence of pleural plaques.

Another survey revealed an Fb-3 increased expression in human mesothelial cells after exposure to FE. Moreover, the Fb-3 levels in the peripheral blood of 40 workers exposed to asbestos were analyzed and compared with those of professionally FE-exposed ones.

Also in this case, results showed Fb-3 higher levels in the FE-exposed group with pleural plaques than in those asbestos-exposed workers who did not show any pleural and/or parenchymal lesions.

At the same time, FE fibers were used to stimulate mesothelial cell cultures. Results showed an Fb-3 hyper-expression after exposure to FE even at low concentrations (see **Figure 5**).

6. Comparative analysis of Fb-3 with other biomarkers

As underlined afore, many surveys focused on researching new MM biomarkers. The reasons of such interest from the scientific community are not purely academic; in fact, even though in several Western countries exposure to asbestos seems to be confined to few professional contexts, in developing countries such as India and China asbestos is still extracted and exploited. For such reason MM continues to be a recurrent disease nowadays, also by reason of a few high-susceptibility population subgroups. About that, it has been demonstrated that hereditary mutations borne by the gene BRCA-associated protein 1 (BAP1) predispose for a higher incidence of some cancers, among which MM.

Several biomarkers have been proposed for diagnosing MM, among them metabolites, proteins and microRNAs (miRNAs). An ideal biomarker ought to spot selectively MM patients from those with other pathologies and/or asbestos-exposed subjects from non-exposed ones. With a view to an early diagnosis and implementation of surveillance programs, the ideal biomarker detection sample would be the blood, for its low invasiveness and better compliance; the pleural liquid would be less ideal, as it requires a more invasive collection technique.

Presently, mesothelin is MM's only and most extensively studied biomarker, recognized by the American Food and Drug Administration (FDA) and by some EU countries. It is a protein precursor with a molecular weight of 71 kDa from whose cleavage, the *megakaryocyte potentiating factor* (MPF), which is then secreted into the blood and the *glycosylated phosphatidylinositol-linked glycoprotein*, a membrane protein, are originated. Physiologically, mesothelin is expressed at a low grade in mesothelial cells and almost in no way in other tissues; its overexpression is instead observed in several forms of cancer, such as MM, ovaric, lung cancer and pancreatic adenomacarcinoma.

Some surveys highlighted the capability to identify MM patients through dosage of SMRPs (*soluble mesothelin-related peptides*) in the serum, getting a 60–90% sensitivity and an 80–85% specificity, as well managing to distinguish between MM subjects, asbestos-exposed ones, nonexposed subjects, and others with benign pleural pathologies. Other experiments showed the possibility to differentiate, through SMRPs serum values, MM patients from those with pleural secondary metastases. Studies on humans assessed SMRPs' dosage in the pleural exudate (PE-SMRPs), reporting higher sensitivity values than those serum-obtained in spotting MM patients.

A metanalysis compared data coming from 12 studies, basing itself on a total of 717 subjects suffering from mesothelioma and 2851 controls, among whom were healthy subjects as well as others with pleural pathologies. The results the authors reached showed an overall sensitivity of 64% and a specificity of 89% for the SMRPs measured in the serum.

It seems clear how mesothelin is the main term of comparison to ascertain Fb-3 effectiveness and its possible introduction in MM clinical routine.

A survey conducted by Creaney et al. [12] compared Fb-3 and mesothelin values in the plasma and pleural liquid of 202 subjects. The population examined included MM patients ($n = 82$), patients with benign asbestos-related diseases ($n = 49$), subjects with malignant exudate ($n = 36$), and others with benign exudate [35]. The authors underlined an enhanced diagnostic accuracy of mesothelin compared to Fb-3, both in plasma (AUC = 0.822 vs. 0.671) and in the pleural liquid (AUC = 0.815 vs. 0.588). However, the Fb-3 concentration in the pleural liquid turned out to be a predictive factor for the patient's survival. MM subjects with Fb-3 lower levels in the pleural liquid than the average had significantly longer survival times than those with levels above the average (14.1 vs. 7.9 months). Mesothelin values and other parameters like neutrophil/lynphocite ratio did not appear significantly correlated with the patients' prognosis.

In a survey by Battolla et al., Fb-3 and SMRPs' levels were contextually evaluated in pleural exudate of patients suffering from MM ($n = 33$), benign pleural lesions ($n = 64$) and secondary pleural metasteses ($n = 23$). Samples were analyzed by ELISA, and revealed Fb-3 values similar among MM subjects and the rest of the cohort (geometric mean = 68.1 vs. 66.2 ng/ml; $P = 0.872$) and significantly increased values of SMRPs in MM patients compared with the rest of the group (geometric mean = 14.6 vs. 3.2 nM; $P < 0.001$).

A survey conducted by Napolitano et al. compared HMGB1 values with mesothelin, Fb-3, and osteopontin (OPN) in the blood. The survey population included: a cohort of subjects who had been treated for pleural exudate derived from benign pathologies (n = 13), from MM (n = 22), and other malignant diseases (n = 25); a group of historically asbestos-exposed workers (n = 20); a group of healthy subjects with no documented exposure to asbestos (n = 20). The results of the study revealed that Fb-3 was the molecule with the highest sensitivity in telling MM subjects from those with other pleural pathologies, followed by HMGB1 hyper-acetylated form, by mesothelin and OPN. The authors concluded that the best diagnostic performance could be obtained combining HMGB1 and Fb-3 values.

Generally speaking, most studies in the literature report a better sensitivity of mesothelin compared with Fb-3, both in plasma and pleural liquid. Instead, comparative studies between Fb-3 and other potential MM biomarkers such as OPN and miRNAs are still missing.

7. Conclusions

MM is a fatal form of cancer derived from pleural mesothelial cells. Its etiology usually involves professional and/or environmental exposure to asbestos. Unluckily, early symptoms of this pathology are commonly nonspecific, and this generally entails a diagnosis of the disease at an advanced stage. There are several studies in literature dealing with potential biomarkers for MM early diagnosis and its differentiation from secondary pleural metastases, benign exudative forms and pleural plaques typical of subjects previously exposed to asbestos. If one considers what said so far, it appears clear that the use of reliable biomarkers (sensitive and specific) might be decisive for MM patients' diagnosis, lengthening their life expectations.

The results of the various studies suggest that Fb3 may have a role in developing neoplastic as well as non-neoplastic diseases of the respiratory tract in subjects exposed to asbestos and/or asbestiform fibers. Moreover, some surveys are looking into the hypothesis that Fb-3 might be accounted for the malignant mutation of mesothelial cells after exposure to asbestos fibers.

In fact, chronic inflammation may induce cancer through the production of several cytokines and growth factors, which, as a consequence, may cause the apoptosis and cell proliferation process to alter. About this, it has been observed that p27, an onco-suppressor gene, often deactivated in tumors, gets downregulated in mesothelial cells after exposure to asbestiform fibers. In the same way, Fb-3 has been seen as significantly decreasing in several cancers, this suggesting its potential role as onco-suppressor gene and as antagonist to angiogenesis. However, conflicting scientific data point out a different role for Fb-3, like a "Dr Jekyll and Mr. Hyde" pattern, and suggest that Fb-3 may rather act as promoter of tumor invasion and survival, as in malignant gliomas, fostering angiogenesis. A reasonable interpretation of such pattern may be due to the aberrant methylation of Fb-3 promoter, since the Fb-3 expression is regulated by the hypermethylation of the promoter and/or by the interference of Fb-3 with the activation of kinase B protein (AKT).

In conclusion, circulating Fb-3 seems to be able to tell healthy asbestos-exposed subjects from MM patients. Fb-3 in the pleural liquid is thought to further differentiate MM subjects from those with benign and/or malignant effusions.

To validate present results and test the effectiveness of Fb-3 combination with other possible biomarkers, it will be necessary to recruit larger numbers of patients.

The combined use of more biomarkers seems likely to guarantee more reliable results in terms of sensitivity and specificity so as to allow to tell, already at an early stage, MM from other pathologies of various nature. In the same way, using several biomarkers together with clinical-diagnostic exams, might contribute to carrying out the screening of populations exposed to asbestos/asbestiform fibers like in the abovementioned case of subjects living in Biancavilla (CT), exposed to FE fibers released in the surrounding area.

Author details

Venerando Antonio Rapisarda* and Caterina Ledda
Coccupational Medicine, Department of Clinical and Experimental Medicine, University of Catania, Catania, Sicily, Italy

*Address all correspondence to: dottore.rapisarda@gmail.com

References

[1] Rapisarda V, Salemi R, Marconi A, Loreto C, Graziano AC, Cardile V, et al. Fluoro-edenite induces fibulin-3 overexpression in non-malignant human mesothelial cells. Oncology Letters. 2016;**12**(5):3363-3367

[2] Rapisarda V, Caltabiano R, Musumeci G, Castrogiovanni P, Ferrante M, Ledda C, et al. Analysis of fibulin-3 after exposure to asbestos-like fibers. Environmental Research. 2017;**156**:381-387

[3] Pass HI, Levin SM, Harbut MR, et al. Fibulin-3 as a blood and effusion biomarker for pleural mesothelioma. The New England Journal of Medicine. 2012;**367**:1417-1427

[4] Jiang Z, Shen W, Ying S, Gao Z, Lou J. Overexpression of fibulin-3 in tumor tissue predicts poor survival of malignant mesothelioma patients from hand-spinning asbestos exposed area in eastern China. Scientific Reports. 2020 Nov 23;**10**(1):20373

[5] Hassan MH, Abuhamdah S, Abdel-Bary M, Wahman M. Circulating and local nuclear expression of survivin and fibulin-3 genes in discriminating benign from malignant respiratory diseases: Correlation analysis. Bioscience Reports. 2021;**41**(1):BSR20203097

[6] Caltabiano R, Loreto C, Vitale E, Matera S, Miozzi E, Migliore M, et al. Fibulin-3 immunoexpression in malignant mesothelioma due to fluoro-edenite: A preliminary report. Future Oncology. 2018;**14**(6s):53-57

[7] Jiang Z, Ying S, Shen W, Shen JW, Tong Y, Zhang X, et al. Plasma Fibulin-3 as a potential biomarker for patients with Asbestos-related diseases in the Han population. Disease Markers. 2017;**2017**:1725354

[8] Battolla E, Canessa PA, Ferro P, Franceschini MC, Fontana V, Dessanti P, et al. Comparison of the diagnostic performance of Fibulin-3 and mesothelin in patients with pleural effusions from malignant mesothelioma. Anticancer Research. 2017;**37**(3):1387-1391

[9] Napolitano A, Pellegrini L, Dey A, et al. Minimal asbestos exposure in germline BAP1 heterozygous mice is associated with deregulated inflammatory response and increased risk of mesothelioma. Oncogene. 2016;**35**:1996-2002

[10] Kirschner MB, Pulford E, Hoda MA, Rozsas A, van Zandwijk N, Klebe S, et al. Fibulin-3 levels in malignant pleural mesothelioma are associated with prognosis but not diagnosis. British Journal of Cancer. 2015;**113**(6):963-969

[11] Kaya H, Demir M, Taylan M, Sezgi C, Tanrikulu AC, Yilmaz S, et al. Fibulin-3 as a diagnostic biomarker in patients with malignant mesothelioma. The Asian Pacific Journal of Cancer Prevention (APJCP). 2015;**16**(4):1403-1407

[12] Creaney J, Dick IM, Meniawy TM, et al. Comparison of fibulin-3 and mesothelin as markers in malignant mesothelioma. Thorax. 2014;**69**:895-902

[13] Corradi M, Goldoni M, Alinovi R, et al. YKL-40 and mesothelin in the blood of patients with malignant mesothelioma, lung cancer and asbestosis. Anticancer Research. 2013;**33**:5517-5524

[14] Lecka-Czernik B, Lumpkin CK Jr, Goldstein S. An overexpressed gene transcript in senescent and quiescent human fibroblasts encoding a novel

protein in the epidermal growth factor-like repeat family stimulates DNA synthesis. Molecular and Cellular Biology. 1995;**15**:120-128

[15] Stone EM, Lotery AJ, Munier FL, Heon E, Piguet B, Guymer RH, et al. A single EFEMP1 mutation associated with both Malattia Leventinese and Doyne honeycomb retinal dystrophy. Nature Genetics. 1999;**22**:199-202

[16] Luo R, Zhang M, Liu L, Lu S, Zhang CZ, Yun J. Decrease of fibulin-3 in hepatocellular carcinoma indicates poor prognosis. PLoS One. 2013;**8**(8):e70511

[17] Nandhu MS, Hu B, Cole SE, Erdreich-Epstein A, Rodriguez-Gil DJ, Viapiano MS. Novel paracrine modulation of notch-DLL4 signaling by fibulin-3 promotes angiogenesis in high-grade gliomas. Cancer Research. 2014;**74**(19):5435-5448

[18] McLaughlin PJ, Bakall B, Choi J, Liu Z, Sasaki T, Davis EC, et al. Lack of fibulin-3 causes early aging and herniation, but not macular degeneration in mice. Human Molecular Genetics. 2007;**16**:3059-3070

[19] Hu B, Thirtamara-Rajamani KK, Sim H, Viapiano MS. Fibulin-3 is uniquely upregulated in malignant gliomas and promotes tumor cell motility and invasion. Molecular Cancer Research. 2009;7:1756-1770

[20] Chen X, Meng J, Yue W, Yu J, Yang J, Yao Z, et al. Fibulin-3 suppresses Wnt/β-catenin signaling and lung cancer invasion. Carcinogenesis. 2014;**35**(8):1707-1716

[21] Wang X, Zhang Q, Li C, Qu X, Yang P, Zheng Y. Fibulin-3 has anti-tumorigenic activities in cutaneous squamous cell carcinoma. Journal of Investigative Dermatology. 2019;**139**(8):1798-1808.e5

[22] Hwang CF, Chien CY, Huang SC, Yin YF, Huang CC, Fang FM, et al. Fibulin-3 is associated with tumour progression and a poor prognosis in nasopharyngeal carcinomas and inhibits cell migration and invasion via suppressed AKT activity. The Journal of Pathology. 2010;**222**(4):367-379

[23] Kim IG, Lee JH, Kim SY, Kim JY, Cho EW. Fibulin-3 negatively regulates ALDH1 via c-MET suppression and increases γ-radiation-induced sensitivity in some pancreatic cancer cell lines. Biochemical and Biophysical Research Communications. 2014;**454**(3):369-375

[24] Li J, Qi C, Liu X, Li C, Chen J, Shi M. Fibulin-3 knockdown inhibits cervical cancer cell growth and metastasis in vitro and in vivo. Scientific Reports. 2018;**8**(1):10594

[25] Wang S, Zhang D, Han S, Gao P, Liu C, Li J, et al. Fibulin-3 promotes osteosarcoma invasion and metastasis by inducing epithelial to mesenchymal transition and activating the Wnt/β-catenin signaling pathway. Scientific Reports. 2017;7(1):6215

[26] Han AL, Veeneman BA, El-Sawy L, Day KC, Day ML. Fibulin-3 promotes muscle-invasive bladder cancer. Oncogene. 2017;**36**(37):5243-5251

[27] Simsek O, Kocael A, Kemik A, Vatankulu B, Kocael P, Halac M, et al. Decreased preoperative serum fibulin-3 levels in colon cancer patients. European Review for Medical and Pharmacological Sciences. 2015;**19**(21):4076-4080

[28] Tong JD, Jiao NL, Wang YX, Zhang YW, Han F. Downregulation of fibulin-3 gene by promoter methylation in colorectal cancer

predicts adverse prognosis. Neoplasma. 2011;**58**(5):441-448

[29] Tian H, Liu J, Chen J, Gatza ML, Blobe GC. Fibulin-3 is a novel TGF-β pathway inhibitor in the breast cancer microenvironment. Oncogene. 2015;**34**(45):5635-5647

[30] Noonan MM, Dragan M, Mehta MM, Hess DA, Wondisford FE, Bhattacharya M. The matrix protein Fibulin-3 promotes KISS1R induced triple negative breast cancer cell invasion. Oncotarget. 2018;**9**(53): 30034-30052

[31] Chapman A, Mulrennan S, Ladd B, Muers MF. Population based epidemiology and prognosis of mesothelioma in Leeds, UK. Thorax. 2008;**63**:435-439

[32] Sugarbaker DJ, Flores RM, Jaklitsch MT, Richards WG, Strauss GM, Corson JM, et al. Resection margins, extrapleural nodal status, and cell type determine postoperative long-term survival in trimodality therapy of malignant pleural mesothelioma: Results in 183 patients. The Journal of Thoracic and Cardiovascular Surgery. 1999;**117**:54-63

[33] Micolucci L, Akhtar MM, Olivieri F, Rippo MR, Procopio AD. Diagnostic value of microRNAs in asbestos exposure and malignant mesothelioma: Systematic review and qualitative meta-analysis. Oncotarget. 2016;**7**(36):58606-58637

[34] Astoul P, Roca E, Galateau-Salle F, Scherpereel A. Malignant pleural mesothelioma: From the bench to the bedside. Respiration. 2012;**83**:481-493

[35] Carbone M, Kanodia S, Chao A, Miller A, Wali A, Weissman D, et al. Consensus report of the 2015 Weinman international conference on mesothelioma. Journal of Thoracic Oncology. 2016;**11**(8):1246-1262

[36] Demir M, Kaya H, Taylan M, Ekinci A, Yılmaz S, Teke F, et al. Evaluation of new biomarkers in the prediction of malignant mesothelioma in subjects with environmental Asbestos exposure. Lung. 2016;**194**(3):409-417

[37] Agha MA, El-Habashy MM, El-Shazly RA. Role of fibulin-3 in the diagnosis of malignant mesothelioma. Egyptian Journal of Chest Diseases and Tuberculosis. 2014;**105**:63-99

[38] Ledda C, Caltabiano R, Vella F, Matera S, Marconi A, Loreto C, et al. Fibulin-3 as biomarker of malignant mesothelioma. Biomarkers in Medicine. 2019;**13**(10):875-886

[39] Ledda C, Senia P, Rapisarda V. Biomarkers for early diagnosis and prognosis of malignant pleural mesothelioma. The Quest Goes on. Cancers (Basel). 2018;**10**(6):203

Section 3

Treatment of Mesothelioma

Chapter 5

Surgical Management of Malignant Pleural Mesothelioma: From the Past to the Future

Alice Bellini, Beatrice Aramini and Franco Stella

Abstract

Malignant pleural mesothelioma (MPM) is an aggressive malignancy with a poor prognosis, principally caused by a prior asbestos exposure. Up to the present, multimodality protocols including surgery with chemotherapy (CT) and/or radiotherapy (RT) represent the therapeutic gold standard for selected patients (epithelial and early-stage MPM). In this context, the aim of surgery is to accomplish the macroscopic complete resection (MCR). There are two main surgical options to obtain MCR—extrapleural pneumonectomy (EPP) and pleurectomy/decortication (PD). The superiority of one surgical approach over the other is still discussed. To date, the decision to carry out one or the other in a multimodal setting is established on surgeons' preference more than on strong scientific evidence. Due to the high morbidity, both surgical techniques should be achieved in tertiary referral centres. In summary, surgery, CT, and RT have failed as single modality therapies with no effects on patients survival. This aspect may be justified by the lack of randomized trials. Thus, novel therapeutic strategies, such as multimodality treatment and targeted agents, seem to prolong the survival and the quality of life. The aim of this chapter is to provide a complete overview of the current surgical approaches to MPM, discussing within the frameworks of pre-operative diagnostic evaluation and multimodality oncological treatments.

Keywords: malignant pleural mesothelioma, extrapleural pneumonectomy, pleurectomy/decortication, multimodality treatment, chemotherapy, radiotherapy, target therapy

1. Introduction

MPM is a rare tumor that has become a world health issue due to its poor prognosis and its increasing incidence, largely due to prior asbestos exposure (the latency is about 20–40 years). Median overall survival (OS) is approximately 1 year in patients with MPM, and the 5-year OS rate is about 10% [1]. In recent years, there has been a notable advancement in the comprehension of MPM pathogenesis, leading to new promising drugs and therapeutic schemes [2, 3]. Particularly, recent trials including innovative drugs, such as targeted therapies or immunotherapies, have encouraged MPM patients [4]. Optimal treatment strategy in MPM has not yet been well established, consequently, current guidelines from the British Thoracic Society (BTS) [5], the American Society of Clinical Oncology (ASCO) [6], the National Comprehensive Cancer Network (NCCN) [1] and the European Society for Medical Oncology (ESMO) [7] have examined similar studies but reached different conclusions. Newly, a task force composed of the European Respiratory Society (ERS), the European Society of Thoracic Surgeons (ESTS), the European Association for Cardio-Thoracic Surgery (EACTS) and the European Society for Radiotherapy and Oncology (ESTRO) [8] proposed updated and practical guidelines on routine management of MPM, after a systematic review of the 2009–2018 literature, including new promising therapies and strategies. Up to the present, therapeutic strategies for MPM are still discussed; therefore, with a lack of a homogeneous consensus on this theme, physicians preferred to evaluate every single patient in a multidisciplinary team to adopt the best treatment based on the performance status of the patient and the stage of the tumor.

The current Eighth Edition of tumor, nodes, metastasis (TNM) classification for MPM [1] is reported in **Tables 1** and **2**. As stated in the aforementioned guidelines, at early stages (disease confined to the pleural envelope, without N2 lymph node involvement) with favorable histology (epithelial), a surgical approach with curative intent in a multimodal protocol appears to be indicated to enhance survival and quality of life. Instead, in advanced stages with distant spread palliative or supportive care must be preferred.

Because of the diffuse growth pattern and the lack of surgical margins, microscopic complete resection is theoretically impossible. Thus, a MCR should be the aim of the surgery, even though the optimal cytoreductive procedure is still controversial [9, 10]. There are two main surgical options to obtain MCR—EPP and PD; the superiority of one technique over the other is still debated [11]. Due to the high morbidity, both surgical techniques should be achieved only in tertiary referral centres with a wide experience in thoracic surgery [12]. Generally, surgery achieves only cytoreduction, hence it must be associated with induction CT (iCT) or adjuvant CT (aCT) with or without adjuvant RT (aRT) to achieve better outcomes in terms of survival and control of the disease.

The best combination of these different therapeutic approaches is still a matter of debate [13, 14]. Hence, the aim of this up-to-dated literature review is to provide a complete overview of the current surgical approaches to MPM, discussing within the frameworks of pre-operative diagnostic evaluation and multimodality oncological treatments.

2. Surgery for MPM

2.1 The importance of the MCR in the surgery for MPM

The MPM is characterized by a singular growth along the pleural surface, representing a challenge for its surgical resection to provide a microscopic free margin (R0 resection) avoiding its direct manipulation. Hence, the best surgical result is a MCR with microscopic positive margins (R1 resection) [9, 10, 15, 16]. For this reason, MCR came to be the main principle of surgery for MPM, based on retrospective data

T	***Primary tumor***
TX	Primary tumor can not bed assessed
T0	No evidence of primary tumor
T1	Tumor limited to the ipsilateral pleural with or without the involvement of: • Visceral pleura • Mediastinal pleura • Diaphragmatic pleura
T2	Tumor involving each of the ipsilateral pleural surfaces (parietal, mediastinal, diaphragmatic, and visceral pleura) with at least one of the following features: • Involvement of diaphragmatic muscle • Extension of tumor from visceral pleura into the underlying pulmonary parenchyma
T3	Locally advanced but potentially resectable tumor. Tumor involving all ipsilateral pleural surfaces (parietal, mediastinal, diaphragmatic, and visceral pleura), with at least one of the following features: • Involvement of the endothoracic fascia • Extension into the mediastinal fat • Solitary, completely resectable focus of tumor extending into the soft tissues of the chest wall • Nontransmural involvement of the pericardium
T4	Locally advanced technically unresectable tumor. Tumor involving all ipsilateral pleural surfaces (parietal, mediastinal, diaphragmatic, and visceral pleura), with at least one of the following features: • Diffuse extension or multifocal masses of tumor in the chest wall, with or without associated rib destruction • Direct transdiaphragmatic extension of the tumor to the peritoneum • Direct transdiaphragmatic extension of the tumor to the contralateral pleura • Direct transdiaphragmatic extension of the tumor to mediastinal organs • Direct transdiaphragmatic extension of the tumor to the spine • Tumor extending through to the internal surface of the pericardium with or without a pericardial effusion; or involving the myocardium
N	***Regional lymph nodes***
NX	Regional lymph nodes can not be assessed
N0	No regional lymph nodes metastases
N1	Metastases in the ipsilateral bronchopulmonary, hilar, or mediastinal (including the internal mammary, peridiaphragmatic, pericardial fat pad, or intercostal) lymph nodes
N2	Metastases in the contralateral mediastinal, ipsilateral, or contralateral supraclavicular lymph nodes
M	***Distant metastasis***
M0	No distant metastasis
M1	Distant metastasis present

TNM: tumor nodes metastasis; MPM: malignant pleural mesothelioma.

Table 1.
Definitions for TNM for MPM (according to the current eighth edition).

showing longer survival for MCR when compared to R2 resection [15, 17, 18]. As claimed by the literature, 30% of the patients addressed to surgery is found unresectable in the operating room [15]. Basically, it is important to improve the preoperative identification of an unresectable disease to prevent a futile explorative thoracotomy (ET), promote enrolment to medical therapies, and avoid expensive and not necessary costs [19].

Stage	T	N	M
IA	T1	N0	M0
IB	T2–T3	N0	M0
II	T1–T2	N1	M0
IIIA	T3	N1	M0
IIIB	T1–T3 T4	N2 Any N	M0 M0
IV	Any T	Any N	M1

MPM: malignant pleural mesothelioma; TNM: tumor nodes metastasis.

Table 2.
Prognostic group for MPM (according to the current eighth edition).

2.2 The pre-operative role of computed tomography (CT) and spirometry

Across the literature, the most common factor precluding MCR is the diffuse chest wall invasion (DCWI), which is frequently associated with the contraction of the ipsilateral hemithorax in the CT scan [15, 20]. Growing up, MPM conducts to a restrictive syndrome and reduces the thoracic cage expansion and the diaphragmatic contraction, leading to a respiratory pump failure, as a necessary consequence [21, 22].

Recently, few authors analyzed the thoracic cage volume (TCV), the aerated lung volumes and the pleural thickness according to Response Evaluation Criteria in Solid Tumors (RECIST) modified criteria (the radiological parameters that correlated with the contracted hemithorax) and the pulmonary functions tests (PFTs), particularly the total lung capacity (TLC) (an indicator of the restrictive syndrome), as possible preoperative predictors of unresectability. Particularly, Burt et al. created a novel three-dimensional radiographic metric of the TCV, based on a fully manual segmentation, and demonstrated that a 5% decrease in TCV compared with the contralateral side was significantly associated with unresectability due to DCWI [15], while Bellini and co-workers used two methods already codified in the literature: the semi-automated segmentation of the aerated lung volumes [23] and the RECIST modified criteria measuring pleural thickness (the sum of the two maximum tumor thicknesses, perpendicular to the chest wall or mediastinum, measured at three levels, was reported as the disease burden) [24]. The Italian group found the TLC and the disease burden as independent predictors of unresectability in the multivariable analysis, with an optimal cut-off value of <77.5% and >120.5 mm, respectively; whereas the aerated lung volumes were significantly associated with ET only in the univariable analysis, probably due to the strong correlation with the disease burden. The PFTs seems to be an additional tool to better improve the preoperative identification of MPM disease not amenable to MCR [20], besides to be indicators of cytoreductive efficacy of iCT, as previously demonstrated by Marulli and collaborators [21, 22]. Moreover, both lung volumes and pleural thickness according to RECIST modified criteria play an important and consolidated prognostic role in MPM survival [23–28]. In particular, the pleural thickness has been recently reported as a useful prognostic indicator of MPM —there is joint approval of the Eighth Edition of the tumor, node and metastasis (TNM) staging system and a recommendation to prospectively evaluate the importance of tumor volume or an approximation by tumor thickness [27–30].

2.3 Surgical indications

Early stages MPM (stage I to IIIA according to Eighth Edition TNM staging system) in patients with epithelial subtype and good performance status represents the best indication for surgery. Conversely, absolute contraindications are patients with sarcomatoid or sarcomatoid-predominant histology, pN2 disease (according to Eighth Edition TNM staging system) and/or stage IV, unless in the context of clinical trials [1, 8, 30, 31]. Despite the overall poor prognosis of biphasic histology, according to recent multicentre analyses, a multimodal approach, including cancer-directed surgery, seems to be associated with improved long-term results in very selected patients with biphasic MPM [31, 32], mostly in patients with a lower proportion of sarcomatoid disease [33]. The ipsilateral nodal disease is not an absolute contraindication for surgery, in fact, the pattern of lymphatic drainage of the pleura does not follow the same pathway as for the lung parenchyma; mediastinal nodes may be the initial site of metastases before the lung parenchyma is involved. The International Association for the Study of Lung Cancer (IASLC) staging project recently reported no survival difference between traditional pN1 and pN2. Therefore, clinical and pathological N1 and N2 are combined into a single N1 category including all ipsilateral, intrathoracic nodal metastases, conversely, contralateral or all extrathoracic nodal metastases (N2 category) represent an absolute contraindication for surgery [34]. Before radical surgery, it is recommended to have a diagnosis not only based on cytology, because of the high risk of diagnostic error, but also on tissue confirmation by pleural biopsy (by either video-assisted thoracoscopy (VATS) or by mini-thoracotomy in the presence of fused pleural space, minimizing the number and size of incisions due to the risk of recurrence in the port-sites) to confirm the presence of microscopic subpleural fat tissue invasion and to allow for adequate immunohistochemical analysis [30].

2.4 Surgical procedures with curative intent: EPP vs. PD, which one to choose?

To obtain MCR there are two main surgical options with curative intent—EPP and PD. Both often allows to obtain only cytoreduction, hence surgical resection must be incorporated in multimodality regimens which include CT and/or RT in the neoadjuvant or adjuvant setting, to achieve better outcomes in term of survival and control of the disease [12, 13]. The EPP is a well-standardized procedure, based on the en bloc resection of the parietal and visceral pleura, ipsilateral lung, pericardium, and hemidiaphragm [35]; it has been deemed for many decades the best technique to achieve MCR with its survival benefits [9]. Conversely, PD is a lung-sparing approach, first reported in 1975 [36] and not yet homogenized in all centres: its description has changed according to the surgical technique, curative intent, and clinical indications [37]. Originally, it was suggested as a cytoreductive substitute in patients with a reduced cardiorespiratory reserve, which cannot tolerate the resection of the entire lung. In 2011, the International Mesothelioma Interest Group (IMIG) and the IASLC recommended that surgical procedures for MPM should be classified into three categories—(1) extended PD (EPD), (2) PD, and (3) partial pleurectomy [38], while mediastinal node sampling should be performed with a goal to obtain at least three nodal stations [1].

Both EPP and EPD required diaphragm and pericardial resections and reconstructions. Due to the lack of consistent guidelines, different materials (alloplastic and autologous) and techniques are available according to surgeons' preferences, with the aim to maximize the strength of the patch and to decrease the complications rate. The most frequent complications after diaphragmatic and pericardial reconstructions are the patch dehiscence with abdominal herniation (mostly in the left side), inferior vena cava (IVC) stenosis, cardiac herniation, cardiac tamponade and infection [39].

The most popular material for diaphragmatic reconstruction is the 2 mm-thick expanded polytetrafluroethylene (e-PTFE), often in its dual mesh formulation (with the 2 different surfaces both reduce the adhesion of abdominal organs and facilitate the proliferation of cells in the thoracic side.), fixed with interrupted non-absorbable stitches across the ribs. The use of a synthetic alloplastic material on one hand permits an improvement in resistance, but on the other hand, it is characterized by a non-insignificant risk of infection (2.4%), while the herniation risk oscillates from 3.8–12%, in particular, the left posterior mediastinum represents the area with the highest incidence of patch dehiscence [39]. To reduce the risk of gastric herniation, it may help leave a small rim (maximus 2 cm) of autologous diaphragm next to the aortic arch and oesophagal hiatus to anchor the patch. On the right side, the herniation of the abdominal organs is less common because of the presence of the liver. However, surgeons should pay attention to preventing the IVC stenosis from leaving a short rim of diaphragmatic tissue or fixing the diaphragmatic mesh to the pericardium edge or the pericardium patch [39].

Similar to a diaphragmatic replacement, synthetic patches are preferred for the repair of the pericardium: among the non-permeable group, the most used is the 0.1 mm-thick e-PTFE, while in the permeable group the polyester and polypropylene prosthesis. The patch is generally sutured with interrupted non-absorbable stitches beginning from the deeper posterior part, while in the inferior side it might be fixed to the diaphragmatic mesh increasing the pericardial space. In fact, the purpose of the pericardial reconstruction is to allow a normal cardiac function, preventing tamponade or diastolic dysfunction. It could be helpful both the fenestration of the mesh or its anchorage leaving unfixed it's superior part for the regular outflow of the pericardial fluid in the directions of the pleural space [39].

EPP involves en bloc resection of the visceral and parietal pleura, lung and, if necessary, ipsilateral hemidiaphragm, and pericardium (**Figure 1**). The lung removal allows administrating a higher dose of RT with no risk of radiation pneumonitis, improving the local control of the disease. This procedure was first employed in 1976 [40], becoming the treatment of choice for potentially resectable MPM. In 1999, Sugarbaker and colleagues reported a 5-year OS rate of 46% and a low mortality rate for patients affected by an early stage epithelial MPM, underwent EPP in a multimodal regimen [12]. Subsequently, there have been different series demonstrating a similar trend with a OS of 20–24 months [35, 41]. One decade ago, in a European survey composed of 802 thoracic surgeons, EPP was considered more efficacious than PD and the supplementation with aCT or other associations of multimodal treatments were deemed to enhance the possibility of cure [42]. Nevertheless, its survival advantages, EPP is charged by some disadvantages: it is a debilitating surgical procedure, associated with a morbidity rate of almost 50% and a mortality rate of 5% even in tertiary referral centres, with high expertise in the surgical management of MPM [41].

In particular, it is associated with a reduction in quality of life, a worsening of postoperative cardiorespiratory function, and difficulties in administration, tolerance, and compliance of adjuvant therapy. A single centre trial (Surgery for Mesothelioma After Radiation Therapy, SMART) embraced a novel protocol, consisting in EPP after intensity-modulate radiation therapy (IMRT) (a short hemi-thoracic high dose technique), with good early and long-term results [43]. However, the employment of EPP as part of the multimodal treatment of MPM has been recently debated after the

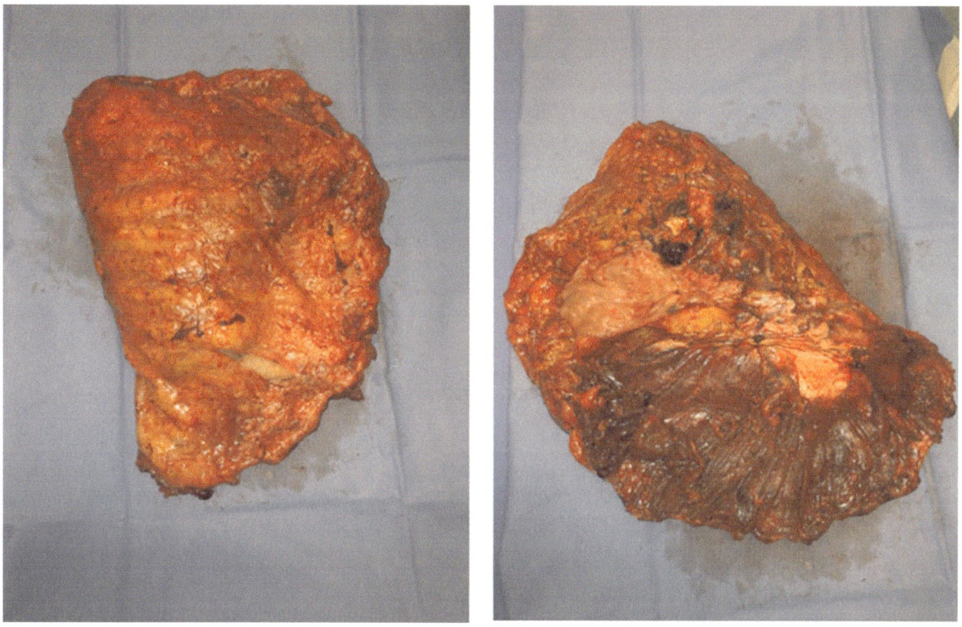

Figure 1.
(a and b) En bloc resection of the lung, parietal, and visceral pleural with diaphragm and pericardium after extrapleural pneumonectomy.

Mesothelioma and Radical Surgery (MARS)-1 trial reports. This wide randomized trial, comparing EPP with no surgery in terms of survival and quality of life, concluded that "EPP within trimodal therapy offers no benefit and possibly harms patient" [44]. Anyhow, these results were controversial because survival was not the primary outcome of the study, the sample size was small, and the surgical mortality was higher than expected—this trial, in fact, faced several problems in the enrolment of patients with few cases treated by few centres with a not acceptable high mortality rate in the EPP arm that finally conditioned the survival results [45].

PD involves the total resection of both the parietal and visceral pleura, while the lung is spared (**Figure 2**).

As claimed by the IMIG classification, it is categorized in [38]:

- *Extended PD*: the parietal and visceral pleurectomy associated with the resection of the pericardium and/or diaphragm;
- *PD*: the parietal and visceral pleurectomy without the removal of the diaphragm or pericardium;
- *Partial pleurectomy (PP)*: the partial removal of the parietal and/or visceral pleura.

The first employment of pleurectomy for MPM was in 1975 by Martin and collaborators, who reported a median OS of 16 months in a series of 14 patients [36], extended the year later with 33 MPM patients with a median OS of 21 months [46].

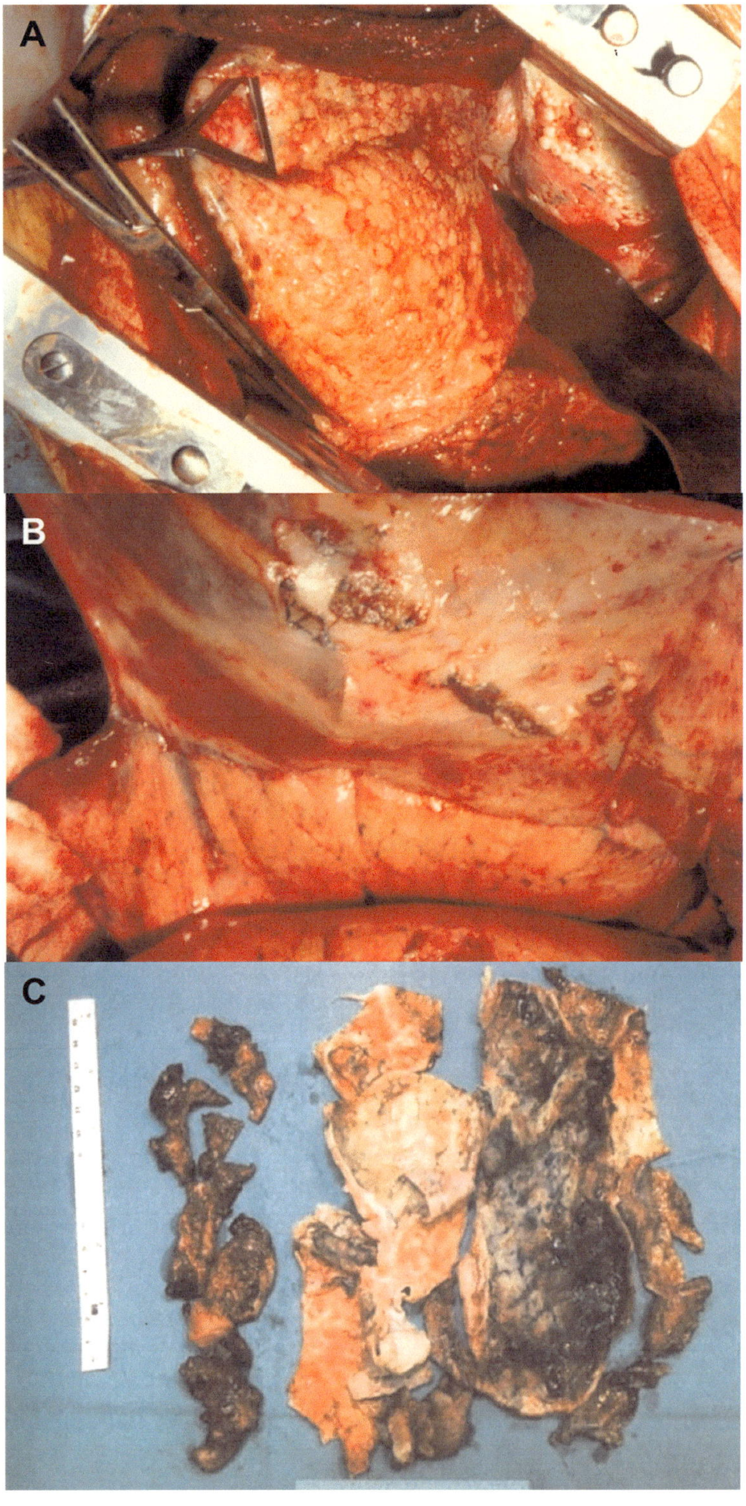

Figure 2.
(A and B) Pleurectomy/decortication (PD). (C) Pathological specimen (visceral and parietal pleura) after PD.

Since then, several non-randomized studies have demonstrated the feasibility and safety of PD with various multimodality schemes involving induction and adjuvant treatments [37, 47, 48]. The preservation of the ipsilateral lung is the main advantage of PD compared to EPP, in fact, it allows a surgical treatment even in patients with a marginal cardiopulmonary reserve, making more feasible adjuvant therapies. The efficacy and radicality of PD in advanced MPM are controversial, however, data from literature are divergent [49]. Almost one decade ago, in an editorial Raja Flores [50] underlined the general trend of thoracic surgeons moving from EPP to PD, due to the lack of solid evidence about a significant survival difference between the aforementioned two surgical procedures [51]. According to the author, the main goal of surgery is the removal of as much tumor as possible preventing pneumonectomy with a consequent reduction in perioperative morbidity and mortality.

On the basis of the currently available data the equation tips in favor of PD rather than EPP. The MARS-2 trial [48], a phase III study of 328 patients with resectable MPM of any sub-type, recently completed the recruitment and, in a little over 2 years, will address the question of whether PD adds any survival benefit to systemic CT alone. While awaiting the results of MARS-2, we are justified in offering surgery as part of multimodality treatment to those with the best prognostic factors, ie, epithelioid with no clinical evidence of nodal disease [30]. The correct surgical strategy must be planned with the intention to accomplish MCR opting for the less invasive technique, basically, surgeons should enter the operating room with the intention to perform PD, except in case of extensive lung invasion. With the lack of randomized controlled trials comparing the two intended to treat techniques, it is still debatable which one provides better long-term outcomes. This is the reason why until now there is not a unique therapeutic approach for MPM and physicians base their decision according to their expertise, the performance status of the patient and the characteristic of the neoplasm. Anyhow, it is important that the sick person and his relatives acquire satisfactory information about both the disease and the available treatments [52].

Among the major complications after both surgical techniques, haemothorax is one of the most frequent, mostly after EPP (1–20.6%) than PD (0–4%). In fact, the extensive pleurectomy and the creation of a post-pneumonectomy cavity increase the risk of bleeding. Surgeons should meticulously verify the hemostasis at the end of the procedure in presence of a normal blood pressure, often using tissue sealants, argon-beam coagulation or oxidized regenerated cellulose products.

Empyema is a frequent complication after surgery for MPM (EPP 1.5–29.7%, PD 4–6.8%), often consequently the development of a bronchopleural fistula (BPF) after EPP (1–12%) in debilitated patients, because of the neoadjuvant treatments and the surgical procedure itself. To prevent the development of such life-threatening complication, it is mandatory keeping the bronchial stump as short as possible, to avoid blind-end secretion retention, and prevent excessive devascularisation of the bronchus. To date, there is no evidence that the preventive use of bronchial stump coverage decreases the rate of BPF after EPP. Late empyema could also occur, several weeks after the intervention, in this case often not associated with BPF.

The peculiar and commonest complication after PD is the prolonged air leakage (3.5–57%), consequently the peeling of the visceral pleura with the underlined lung damage. This kind of complication could also cause an empyema due to ascending infection through the longtime chest drain. Surgeons should carefully reduce the post-operative air leaks, mending the lung with stapling device, sutures and sealant. Most of the time conservative management is a correct strategy with the removal of the active suction as soon as possible and the preservation of the chest tube until the resolution of the air leaks with a satisfactory lung expansion, which may take even 2–3 weeks. The post-operative management after PD is not well standardized among the centres—to prevent bleeding and air leakage, some centres prefer to keep patients on mechanical ventilation with positive and expiratory pressure (up to 48 h) to maintain the maximal lung inflation, which aids both the parietal hemostasis by compression and the closure of the parenchymal wounds; other centres prefer to reduce positive pressure ventilation to minimize the air leaks by extubating the patient as soon as possible [37].

2.5 Extracorporeal life support (ECLS) for life-threatening complications in MPM's surgery: is it worthwhile?

In thoracic surgery, the use of ECLS in the postoperative period is augmented in the last decades [53]. Up to now, the unique absolute contraindication to extracorporeal membrane oxygenation (ECMO) is a pre-existing state incompatible with healing, such as an end-stage tumor [54]. Literature provides only a few reports on ECLS as a bridge to support oncological patients affected by complications of their illness [55], its therapy [56, 57] or cardiac arrest [58]. MPM is a locally aggressive tumor, with a very poor prognosis. The multimodality therapies including surgery offered to selected cases (early stages with epithelial histology) are often characterized by major and/or minor perioperative morbidities [13]. According to Burt et al., the EPP is burdened by a significantly higher rate of acute distress respiratory syndrome (ARDS) (8.4 vs. 0.8%) and 30-day mortality (10.5 vs. 3.1%), compared to the PD [52, 59]. Anyhow, in the case of perioperative complications after surgery for MPM the employment of ECLS represents an ethical dilemma due to the fatal nature of this malignancy.

Fica and collaborators mentioned the use of a single-site veno-venous ECMO to support ventilation in an early post-pneumonectomy broncho-pleural fistula [57], while Bellini and collaborators successfully used the veno-arterial (V-A) ECMO as cardiac support in two MPM patients (66%), conversely, the only case (33%) of V-A ECMO implanted primarily for respiratory support in pneumonia-associated ARDS of the residual lung had a negative outcome [60]. Similar results were reported in the literature; according to Gow and collaborators, patients with a better pulmonary reserve and cardiac indication for ECLS are the better oncological candidates for ECMO [61].

The disease process itself and/or the employed treatments lead patients with thoracic cancer to have less pulmonary reserve compared to adults generally demanding ECLS. Secondary infections and bleeding are the major problems for the use of ECLS for oncological patients [61], both potentially life-threatening. In this scenario, on one hand, we have potentially reversible complications not responsive to conventional therapies, while on the other hand frail and immunosuppressed patients with poor prognosis and at risk to develop life-threatening ECMO-related drawbacks.

In accordance with the aforementioned recent literature, in case of a potentially reversible condition especially if heart-related, ECLS could be used as a stopgap device until common therapies work, in very selected MPM patients, permitting the recovery and the completion of the multimodal protocol [60, 61].

2.6 Palliative surgery

The MesoVATS trial is an open-label randomized controlled trial conducted in 12 centres in the United Kingdom, that compared PP by VATS versus talc pleurodesis in patients with MPM [62]. There were no differences between groups in the OS at 1 year nor at 6 months of follow-up. Furthermore, the benefits of VATS-PP (better quality of life, less short-term pleural effusion) do not balance the inconveniences (surgical complications and longer hospital stay leading to more costs). Guidelines strongly recommend talc poudrage via thoracoscopy to control a recurrent MPM effusion as the first choice to achieve pleurodesis in patients with expanded lungs, while weakly suggest, with a low grade of recommendation, palliative VATS-PP to obtain pleural effusion control in symptomatic patients fit enough to undergo surgery who cannot benefit from (or after the failure of) chemical pleurodesis or indwelling catheter [8].

2.7 Surgery for MPM relapse

Recurrence of MPM after multimodality treatment is a common problem. Nevertheless, there has been no established therapy for relapse to date. Major studies about the treatment of recurrent MPM are reported in **Tables 3** and **4**. Over the literature, MPM with distant spread (associated or not with local relapse) is the most frequent pattern of recurrence, mostly in the EPP group, while the PD group showed a higher local-only failure rate [63–71]. A poor prognosis for recurrent MPM after multimodality treatment has been reported in the literature, with a median post-recurrence survival (PRS) after EPP ranging from 3 to 6.5 months [64–66, 72]. Newly,

Author	Surgery, N	Multimodality, N	Relapse, N (%)	Pattern of recurrence, %
Kostron, 2016 [63]	EPP, 136	Bimodal, 47 Trimodal, 59	106 (77.9)	L 24.3 D 19.9 L + D 33.8
Takuwa, 2017 [64]	EPP, 59	Bimodal, 27 Trimodal, 12	39 (66.1)	NR
Kai, 2018 [65]	EPP, 29 PD, 15	Bimodal, 26 Trimodal, 18	32 (72.7)	L 18.2 D 27.3 L + D 27.3
Soldera, 2019 [66]	EPP, 93	Bimodal 43 Trimodal 10	53 (57.0)	L 5.4 D 38.7 L + D 12.9
Nakamura, 2020 [67]	PD, 90	Bimodal, 90	57 (63.3)	L 43 D 6.7 L + D 13.3
Politi, 2010 [68]	EPP, 8	NR	8 (100)	L 50 D 50
Okamoto, 2013 [69]	EPP, 10	NR	8 (80)	L 40 D 40
Burt, 2012 [70]	EPP, 32 PD, 15	NR	47 (100)	L 100
Bellini, 2021 [71]	EPP, 49 PD, 45	Bimodal, 18 Trimodal, 76	94 (100)	L, 28.7 D, 28.7 L + D, 42.6

MPM: malignant pleural mesothelioma; EPP: extrapleural pneumonectomy; PD: pleurectomy/decortication; NR: not reported; L: local; D: distant; L + D: local+distant.

Table 3.
Major studies about the treatment of recurrent MPM: Multimodality regimen and pattern of failure.

Author	Median DFS (m)	Relapse treatment, N (%)	Median PRS (m)	Median OS (m)
Kostron, 2016 [63]	9	None, 28 (26.4) Surgery, 16 (15.1) Medical treatment, 73 (68.9)	7	22[a]
Takuwa, 2017 [64]	11.6	None, 12 (30.7) Medical treatment, 27 (69.2)	6.5	22
Kai, 2018 [65]	Overall, 14[b] EPP, 13[b] PD, 21[b]	Medical treatment, 17 (53.1)	Overall, 5 EPP, 3 PD, 20	Overall, 22[b] EPP, 17[b] PD, 34[b]
Soldera, 2019 [66]	NR	None, 27 (50.9) Medical treatment, 15 (28.3) NR, 11 (20.8)	4.8	NR
Nakamura, 2020 [67]	19	Surgery, 3 (5.3) Medical treatment, 40 (70.2) Best supportive care, 14 (24.5)	14.4	57[b]
Politi, 2010 [68]	NR	Surgery, 8 (100)	14.5	NR
Okamoto, 2013 [69]	15.4	Surgery, 2 (25) Medical treatment, 6 (75)	17.8	49.6
Burt, 2012 [70]	16.1	Surgery, 47 (100)	Epithelial, 20.4 Biphasic, 7.0	44.9
Bellini, 2021 [71]	Overall, 14 EPP, 20 PD, 11	None, 13 (13.8) Surgery, 13 (13.8) Medical treatment, 68 (72.3)	Overall, 12 EPP, 14 PD, 8	Overall, 33 EPP, 38 PD, 23

MPM: malignant pleural mesothelioma; EPP: extrapleural pneumonectomy; PD: pleurectomy/decortication; NR: not reported; L: local; D: distant; L + D: local+distant; DFS: disease-free survival; PRS: post recurrence survival; OS: overall survival, calculated from the date of surgery, except (a) from the first cycle of neoadjuvant chemotherapy; (b) from the date of pleural biopsy.

Table 4.
Major studies about the treatment of recurrent MPM: Oncological outcomes.

comfortable PRS were described after PD by Nakamura et al. and Kai and collaborators (14.4 and 20 months, respectively) [65, 67].

Conversely, Bellini and collaborators recently noted that the type of surgical resection did not affect the PRS (14 and 8 months in the EPP and PD group, respectively) if patients are fit enough to receive post-recurrence treatments [71]. Across the literature, the post-recurrence treatment is the main predictor of better PRS [63, 65, 67], in particular, Bellini and co-authors found tailored medical therapies as the best strategy to face relapse, even in the case of local failure [71], in contrast with satisfactory PRS after redoing surgery, which was reported by Kostron et al. [63]. The Italian group cautiously hypothesized that the early local-only failure may likely reflect a less radical local resection that could benefit from timely systemic therapies, rather than redo surgery that is rarely radical in most of the cases [71]. Moreover, several authors reported a long disease-free survival (DFS) (≥12 months) as significantly associated with good survival [61, 67, 71], probably reflecting a slower tumor growth speed associated with a less aggressive recurrent disease. Furthermore, epithelial histology [65, 71] and local recurrence [71] resulted as a favorable prognostic factor for PRS, the latter may be due to a less deleterious effect on performance status and, consequently, on survival compared with distant spread [71]. In conclusion, in patients presenting with recurrence of MPM after an MCR procedure, radical surgery to resect the recurrent tumor could have a role in the improvement of survival in selected patients [73].

3. Multimodality treatment for MPM

3.1 Bimodal and trimodal therapy in MPM

The microscopic complete resection represents an unattainable goal for surgery alone in MPM disease. For this reason, in the last decades, the surgical approach is mainly used as cytoreduction with improved survival, but with the necessity at least to combine with a bimodal/trimodal treatment, although the income of the novel strategies as immunotherapy, are suggesting a multimodal approach [40, 62, 74, 75]. The debate regarding the possible surgical approach as the closest to the radicality for MPM is still opened [76, 77]. In particular, the believers for EPP as the most oncologically correct approach, strongly support the theory that a near-complete surgical resection associated with chemo-or high-dose aRT may be the best treatment for earlier stages [78]. Recent studies have shown improved survival with EPP associated with neoadjuvant or adjuvant chemoradiotherapy [79], in highly-selected patients, although this type of surgery is very aggressive and invasive and not far from postoperative complications with significant morbidity (25%) and mortality (4–15%) [5]. In 2011 the MARS-1 trial compared patients treated with EPP and patients without, defining this surgery as not effective for the high morbidity and 30-day mortality. Particularly, it was a feasibility multicentre randomized controlled trial carried on between October 2005 and November 2008 in 12 English Hospitals. It included 112 patients aged 18 years or older affected by MPM and fit enough to undergo trimodal treatment. In the pre-randomization registration phase, all patients underwent induction platinum-based CT, followed by a clinical revaluation. The main reasons for not proceeding to randomization were a progression of the disease (33 patients), inoperability (five patients), and patient choice (19 patients). Finally, 50 patients were randomly assigned (1:1): 24 to EPP followed by radical RT and 26 to no EPP. The EPP was completed in 16 patients (in five patients it was not started and in three it was abandoned). The clinical outcomes evaluated were the proportion of patients of the EPP group who completed the trimodal treatment; perioperative mortality; quality of life; OS; and disease-free survival. Of the 16 surgical treated patients, there were tw perioperative deaths, while eight completed the trimodal protocol receiving the radical RT. Serious adverse events were higher in the EPP group (n = 10) than in the no EPP group (n = 2). The median OS for the EPP and the no EPP group were 14.4 months and 19.5 months, respectively. The median DFS for the EPP and the no EPP group were 7.6 months and 9 months, respectively. There was a statistically significant difference in the survival outcomes, while a trend toward a lower quality of life in the EPP group was reported.

Following the MARS-1 trial, the scientific community and surgeons focused their attention on PD, which is for sure less invasive than EPP, but not less effective than EPP [80, 81]. In particular, in the last decades, some retrospective studies and systematic reviews described a comparable survival between the two procedures, but with less morbidity and mortality for the patients treated with PD [51, 74, 82–85] with the association of improved quality of life [84–86], although there are also research groups showing no difference in morbidity and mortality [87–89]. For the fact that data are still extremely different [90], the most focused expert for MPM suggests that a multidisciplinary approach and randomized controlled trials need to be set to further define the best surgery in MPM [42, 90–94]. In particular, the MARS-2 trial is trying to set if PD plus iCT may offer an improvement of the survival than the only CT [48, 91, 95]. Regarding the most updated recommendation, several scientific societies use a trimodal approach (surgery, CT and RT) for MPM) [1, 6, 7, 96]. This has been also confirmed by the BTS and the European Respiratory Society for clinical trials [5, 97]; although the timing for this therapy is still unknown as well as also the sequences of each treatment [97]. However, even in the case of the trimodal approach, the long-term survival of these patients remains still poor and only 5% survive at 5 years [98]. The association of pemetrexed (folate antimetabolite) plus B12 and folic acid supplementation [1, 5–7, 97] is an association with the most standard platinum-based therapy, cisplatin, typically, or carboplatin [99, 100], seems to improve the survival by 2.8 months compared with single drug treatment, probably for the fact that B12 and folic acid supplementation reduce the toxicity, especially in elderly patients [101]. In a recent large phase III trial, MAPS, even the use of bevacizumab, a vascular endothelial growth factor (VEGF) inhibitor in combination with pemetrexed/cisplatin is strongly recommended, which compares pemetrexed/cisplatin alone [102]. In particular, this trial showed improved survival of 2.7 months in unresectable MPM [102]. The ASCO has suggested vinorelbine as second-line treatment, although the NCCN suggested immunotherapy and CT as second-line treatment [1]. In particular, the second-line pemetrexed seems to have some effect against tumor, reducing the tumor progression, as described in a phase III trial [103]; for vinorelbine, the recent randomized controlled trials showed improved survival in patients treated with this drug [104] with good control of symptoms. There are other treatments as PD with intraoperative intracavitary hyperthermic CT, although more studies need to support and analyze concerning the long-term results [105–113]. The majority of studies that evaluate the trimodal approach are retrospective reviews [114–119]. Since 2007, a multicentric clinical trial demonstrated that iCT plus EPP is feasible [41] showing an OS of 23 months compared with patients not treated with surgery with a survival of 19.8 months [41]. An Italian study published similar results [120]. The combination with neoadjuvant cisplatin/pemetrexed treatment has been discussed since 2009 in a multicentric phase II clinical trial in which patients in stage I-III MPM underwent 4 cycles of cisplatin/pemetrexed. Of these patients, who showed a good response to this medical treatment has been then underwent EPP followed by adjuvant hemithoracic radiation [121] with a median survival of 29.1 months with a 2-year survival of 61.2% [122]. These data let the researcher to conclude that a trimodal therapy may be effective and beneficial [122]. In 2010 the European Organization for Research and Treatment of Cancer (EORTC) published a similar multicentre phase II study [121], in which 65% of the patients underwent EPP 65% plus aRT showed a good result for the 42% of patients, although the neoadjuvant therapy associated with EPP, and adjuvant therapy have been shown to be challenging for the poor long term results [41, 116–119]. With regards to the less invasive surgical treatment in MPM, represented by PD, few studies considered the use of trimodal therapy with PD. In particular, in 2012, a non-randomized prospective trial compared EPP to PD in trimodal approach [82] comparing 3 cycles of either cisplatin/gemcitabine or cisplatin/pemetrexed before EPP and aRT to PD with hyperthermic pleural lavage with povidone-iodine and aCT [82]. However, the median survival was 12.8 months for

EPP patients, although a better survival of 23 months has been noted for the second group of patients. These results demonstrated that PD is a more feasible approach with better outcomes for MPM patients underwent trimodal therapy [82]. The role of adjuvant or neoadjuvant radiation therapy is not yet been clarified. In particular, the classic hemithoracic radiation of the entire pleural cavity after EPP is not a problem [123], although the lungs and the other organs cannot be spared from the radiation [124]. However, recent retrospective studies have shown an increased local recurrence in patients treated with adjuvant IMRT following EPP [125]. Recently, the SMART trial concluded the analysis about the role of neoadjuvant IMRT in T1–3N0 MPM followed by EPP, associated with aCT (cisplatin and an anti-folate) in case of mediastinal lymph nodes involvement, achieving encouraging survival results. The results were satisfying in consideration of a median OS of 42.8 months for the epithelial subtype, compared with 18 months for the biphasic one. The authors postulated that a probable mechanism for the distant spread is the spillage of the tumor cells into the coelomic cavities during EPP, hence the IMRT immediately before surgery could inactive these cells making them non-viable, preventing distant seeding with better survival outcomes. Probably the epithelial subtype is more sensible to the action of IMRT. Possible confounder factors for these promising survival results may be as follow: firstly, the criteria for inclusion in the trial were strict leading to a possible selection bias, secondly, the presence of BAP1 mutations (associated with better OS regardless of therapy) was not routinely investigated, so the potential inclusion of these patients in the trial could confound. [43]. In 2016 a group from Memorial Sloan Kettering Cancer Centre (MSKCC) showed the feasibility of IMRT and iCT and PD in IMPRINT phase II trial [126]; however, the same researcher's group published a retrospective study comparing PD trimodal therapy with conventional RT to hemithoracic IMRT [126] with better survival for the patients treated with IMRT [127]. In US both ASCO and NCCN- guidelines strongly support the multimodality treatment for stages I-III epithelioid MPM [128]. The upcoming MARS-2 results may be very helpful to clarify the feasibility and benefits of the multimodality treatment [128]. **Table 5** summarizes the main studies commented on in this paragraph.

3.2 New target therapies in MPM

Although the scientific community is studying genes and proteins which may be used to set new treatments against MPM, the targets for mesothelioma have not been clearly yet identified. Besides the fact that the common MPM treatments including surgery, CT and radiation therapies show a poor OS from 9 to 17 months from the diagnosis [120, 129, 130], new emerging treatments are setting from the scientific community to improve the quality of life and the survival. The most used approach in this field is immunotherapy which seems to play an important role in MPM for the connections and reactions with the patient immunity, driving immunoregulatory mechanisms with a direct good response [131, 132]. In particular, in patients with MPM showing a high infiltrate of cytotoxic CD8+ T associated with programmed death-ligand 1 (PDL-1) expression, the use of pembrolizumab and nivolumab, or nivolumab with the cytotoxic T lymphocyte antigen 4 (CTLA-4) antibody ipilimumab showed very encouraging results [133, 134].

Several trials have been published showing the use of *immunotherapy* in advanced MPM alone or with standard CT. In particular, pembrolizumab seems to improve by 22%, the response rate compared with gemcitabine or vinorelbine which showed a 6% of response [135]. However, other immunotherapies have been analyzed in the last

Author, year, type of study	Type of surgery, N	Multimodal treatment, N	Median OS (m)
Spaggiari L, 2014, multicentre retrospective [79]	EPP, 518	iCT, 271 aRT, 213 aCT, 43 aRT+aCT, 117	18
Fahrner R, 2012, single centre retrospective [98]	EPP, 21	Port-site RT, 18 iCT, 19: platinum+gemcitabine, 15 platinum+pemetrexed, 4 aRT, 16	707 days
Katirtzoglou N, 2010, multicentre phase II [100]	Unresectable, 62	CT with carboplatin+pemetrexed	14
Zalcman G, 2016, multicentre randomized controlled open-label phase III [102]	Unresectable, 448	Cisplatin+bevacizumab, 223 Cisplatin only, 225	With bevacizumab: 18.8 Cisplatin only: 16.1
Muers MF, 2008, multicentre randomized [104]	Unresectable, 409	ASC alone (treatment could include steroids, analgesics drugs, bronchodilatators, palliative radiotherapy), 136 ASC plus mitomycin+vinblastine +cisplatin, 137 ASC plus vinorelbine, 136	ASC alone: 7.6 ASC plus CT: 8.5
Burt BM, 2018, single centre phase I [107]	EPP, 59 PD, 41 Debulking, 4	HIOC with gemcitabine added to cisplatin, 104 aCT, 45 aRT, 10	All 20.3 EPP 17.7 PD 38.8
Opitz I,. 2020, single centre phase I [109]	PD, 12	Intracavitary cisplatin-fibrin, 12	21
Ried M,. 2013, single centre prospective observational [111]	PD, 10	HIOC with cisplatin, 10	NR
Sugarbaker DJ, 2013, single centre retrospective [113]	EPP, 74 (53 HIOC group) PD, 29 (19 HIOC group)	HIOC with cisplatin, 72 No HIOC, 31	HIOC: 35.3 No HIOC: 22.8
Rusch VW, 2001, single centre phase II [114]	EPP, 62 PD, 5	aRT, 57 (54 EPP; 3 PD)	EPP: 17 Early stages 33.8 Advanced stages 10
de Perrot M, 2009, single centre retrospective [116]	EPP, 45 Unresectable, 15	iCT: Cisplatin+vinorelbine, 26 Cisplatin+pemetrexed, 24 Cisplatin+raltitrexed, 6 Cisplatin+gemcitabine, 4 aRT, 30	Trimodality completed 59
Thieke C, 2015, single centre retrospective [118]	EPP, 62	iCT, 62 cisplatin+pemetrexed, 30 carboplatin+pemetrexed, 23 cisplatin+gemcitabine, 9 aRT (IMRT), 62	20.4

Author, year, type of study	Type of surgery, N	Multimodal treatment, N	Median OS (m)
Rea F, 2007, single centre prospective [120]	EPP, 17	iCT with carboplatin+gemcitabine, 21 aRT, 15	All 25.5 EPP, 27.5
Van Schil PE, 2009, multicentre phase II [121]	EPP, 42	iCT with cisplatin+pemetrexed, 55 aRT, 37	All 18.4 Trimodality completed 33
Krug LM, 2009, multicentre phase II [122]	EPP, 54	iCT, 77 aRT, 40	All 16.8 Trimodality completed 29.1
Cho BC, 2021, single centre phase II	EPP, 96 Epithelial, 83 Biphasic, 8 Unkown, 5	iRT (IMRT), 96	24.4 Epithelial: 42.8 Biphasic:18
Rimner A, 2016, multicentre phase II [126]	PD, 8 Partial pleurectomy, 13 Unresectable, 11	iCT, 45: Cisplatin+pemetrexed, 26 Carboplatin+pemetrexed, 18 Combination, 4 aRT (IMPRINT), 27	Trimodality completed 23.7
Shaikh F, 2016, single centre retrospective [127]	PD, 209	aRT: conventional, 131 IMPRINT, 78 Chemotherapy, 85 (15 conventional, 70 IMPRINT)	Conventional,12.3 IMPRINT, 20.2

OS: overall survival; EPP: extrapleural pneumonectomy; iCT: induction chemotherapy; aRT: adjuvant radiotherapy; aCT: adjuvant chemotherapy; PD: pleurectomy/decortication; ASC: active symptom control; HIOC: heated intraoperative chemotherapy; NR: not reported; iRT: induction radiotherapy; IMPRINT: intensity-modulated pleural radiotherapy; IMRT: intensity-modulated radiotherapy.

Table 5.
Summary of the main studies commented in Section 3.1.

decades, for example, in MAPS2 open-label, phase 2 trial that has been studied in 21 French hospitals aiming to set nivolumab alone or combined with ipilimumab. This study showed a 12-weeks disease control in 44% of patients who received only nivolumab, compared with the 50% who underwent nivolumab plus ipilimumab [130]. In January of this year, the Checkmate 743 study was published in Lancet, which reported the superiority of the combination of nivolumab (3 mg/kg every 2 weeks) + ipilimumab (1 mg/kg every 6 weeks) over the above standard. With a significant advantage in the entire study population, particularly marked in the sarcomatoid subtype [136]. For patients progressing to the first line, however, no scheme has been shown to improve survival; however, these patients can be offered gemcitabine, vinorelbine or rechallenge with pemetrexed mono-CT, with unfortunately marginal benefits. Nivolumab, on the other hand, in a phase 3 study (CONFIRM) conducted against placebo in a heavily pretreated population, has shown efficacy in improving both progression-free survival and OS, but at the moment the drug is not approved in Italy. this indication [137].

From preclinical evidence, the role of angiogenesis in the development of this disease and the potential efficacy of inhibiting this mechanism appears to be relevant, although in lines subsequent to the first some *antiangiogenic drugs* have already been tested without success [138]. In particular, there is a strong rationale for angiogenesis inhibition in mesothelioma. VEGF plays an important role as an autocrine growth factor and strong mitogen in mesothelioma. Furthermore, the abnormal tumor vasculature increases the interstitial pressure and hypoxia, which may hinder the effect of the anticancer drugs against mesothelioma cells. Ramucirumab is a fully humanized monoclonal antibody directed against the VEGF receptor 2 (VEGFR-2), currently reimbursed in Italy for use in clinical practice in gastric cancer and tested in numerous other solid tumors [139]. VEGFR-2 is expressed not only in 90% of mesothelioma cells but also on the surface of macrophages present in the tumor microenvironment, considered to be responsible for the resistance to chemo- and immunotherapeutic treatments [140]. Inhibiting this receptor seems to allow the switch from a hypoxic and treatment-resistant environment to a more sensitive and immuno-permissive tumor milieu. In this context, the RAMES study was born, a multicentre, phase 2, randomized and double-blind trial [141]. In the study, which involved 26 Italian centres, patients with Eastern Cooperative Oncology Group performance status (ECOG PS) 0–2 and diagnosed with progressive MPM during or after a first-line with platinum and pemetrexed were enrolled. Patients were randomized to a second line with gemcitabine 1000 mg/m^2 on days 1 and 8 of every 21 plus placebo (in the control group) or ramucirumab (an anti-VEGFR2 antibody) at 10 mg/m^2 on day 1 of each cycle up to progression or severe toxicity. Central randomization was performed according to a minimization algorithm, using the following stratification factors: ECOG PS, age, histology and time to first-line progression (>/<6 months) [141]. The primary endpoint of the study was OS. Secondary aims were progression-free survival, objective response rate, disease control rate, drug safety, patient quality of life and the possible presence of predictive markers. It was planned to enroll 156 patients to obtain a power of 80% assuming a benefit of the experimental treatment of 13% at 1 year compared to the standard arm. From December 2016 to July 2018, 165 patients were enrolled, of whom 161 were correctly assigned and received treatment, 83 in the placebo arm and 81 in the experimental arm. The median age was 69, with about 40% over seventy in both arms. 74% of patients were male and 99% had an ECOG PS of 0–1 [141]. The database was closed in March 2020 and, after a median follow-up of 21.9 months, the observed OS was higher in the experimental arm (Hazard Ratio 0.71; $p = 0.028$). Specifically, in the ramucirumab arm, the median survival was 13.8 months versus only 7.5 months in the placebo arm and the one-year probability of survival improved from 33 to 56% with the addition of ramucirumab [141]. Progression free survival was also higher in the experimental arm (median 6.4 versus 3.3 months), but without reaching statistical significance ($p = 0.082$). Disease control was achieved in 73% of patients treated in the ramucirumab group versus 52% in the placebo arm [141]. A post hoc analysis showed a duration of response of 8.4 months in the experimental arm versus 5.4 months in the standard arm [141]. The pre-specified analysis of the subgroups shows that the survival advantage was independent of the histological subtype and the time of progression of the tumor to the first line [141]. No unexpected toxicities occurred. Grade 3–4 adverse events were recorded in 44% of patients treated with gemcitabine + ramucirumab compared to 30% in the gemcitabine + placebo arm. In particular, the most frequent severe toxicities were neutropenia (20% and 12% in the experimental and standard arms, respectively), arterial hypertension (6% with ramucirumab, 0 with placebo) and fatigue (5% and 4% respectively) [141]. The authors conclude that the association between ramucirumab and gemcitabine significantly improved the OS of patients with progressive MPM following standard first-line CT, with a favorable safety profile. It is clear, however, that in light of the new standard of treatment with the immunotherapy brace nivolumab + ipilimumab, the scheme proposed by the RAMES study [141] is part of a therapeutic context that has changed from the one that had seen the start of the study: in particular, the scheme gemcitabine—ramucirumab has not been tested in patients who have received the combination of the 2 immunotherapies. In addition, the treatment landscape of pleural mesothelioma may still change, pending the results of randomized trials, following interesting phase 2 data for first-line chemo-immunotherapy (NCT02899195 and NCT04334759). Taking this into account, ramucirumab, given its action not only on cancer cells but also on the immune infiltrate and tumor microenvironment, could continue to play a role in patients progressing to chemo-immunotherapy, but further studies will need to be conducted.

Another important drug is the *CTLA-4 inhibitor* tremelimumab which has been studied in a randomized phase II trial (DETERMINE) in 571 patients with a median survival of 7.7 months compared with patients who underwent placebo with 7.3 months of survival: although its safety profile was consistent, tremelimumab did not significantly improve OS [142].

3.3 T-cell therapies

Adoptive T-cell therapy seems to be promising in MPM and this has been highlighted in a recent phase I trial studying the *chimeric antigen receptor (CAR) T-cell therapy* targeting mesothelin in MPM patients. Of 18 patients treated with a single dose of CD28-costimulated MSLN CAR-T cells plus the I-caspase-9 safety gene treated intrapleurally showed that in 14 patients, 2 had complete remission, 5 partial, and 4 patients showed the stability of the disease [143]. In the context of safety, no CAR-T cell-related toxicities have been noted. The most promising approach seems to be represented by the combination between CAR-T cells and *anti- programmed death-1 (PD-1) therapy* [144], although these considerations need to be further investigated.

3.4 Vaccines

One of the most considered new therapies against MPM is vaccine therapy. In particular, the *Wilms tumor-1 (WT1) protein* in MPM is highly expressed and it is considered a future target for the setting of a cancer vaccine. A recent phase II randomized trial evaluated a WT1 analogue peptide vaccine associated with immunologic adjuvants, showing an improved survival at 1 year (45%) compared with the control group with a 33% of survival rate. However, the OS for vaccinated patients was 22.8 months compared with patients not treated (18.3 months) [145].

Other new target agents as *dendritic cells (DC) therapy* started to be recently considered to investigate the anti-tumor immune response [146, 147].

3.5 Other investigational therapies

Besides the vaccines and the T-cells therapies which are coming up for the better control of MPM, the oncolytic viruses and other targets as some vascular endothelial growth factors receptors (*VEGFR*), the platelet-derived growth factor receptor (*PDGFR*), and the fibroblast growth factor receptor (*FGFR*) tyrosine-kinase inhibitor, are under consideration. Some phase I/II clinical trials are running at the moment to evaluate the safety of the biological effects [148–152].

4. Conclusions

In conclusion, the optimal treatment of MPM is still a matter of debate. Surgery, CT, and RT have failed as single modality therapies with no effects on patients' survival. It is evident that optimal multidisciplinary care is fundamental in the management of MPM patients, as the best results are obtained when patients manage to undergo more complex treatment protocols, often consisting in trimodality approaches. New prospective studies are needed to provide high-quality evidence on the field. While it is reasonable to assume that surgery will remain a central component in the multimodality treatment of MPM, a great development is expected from novel treatment modalities such as targeted therapies, T-cell therapy, vaccines and other investigational therapies, leading to the possibility of prolonged control of the disease, increased survival rates, and better quality of life.

Author details

Alice Bellini[1*], Beatrice Aramini[2] and Franco Stella[2]

1 Division of Thoracic Surgery, Department of Surgery, G.B. Morgagni—L. Pierantoni Hospital, Forlì, Italy

2 Division of Thoracic Surgery, Department of Diagnostic and Specialty Medicine–DIMES of the Alma Mater Studiorum, University of Bologna, G.B. Morgagni–L. Pierantoni Hospital, Forlì, Italy

*Address all correspondence to: alice.bellini@auslromagna.it

References

[1] National Comprehensive Cancer Network (NCCN). Malignant Pleural Mesothelioma Guidelines Version 2.2021—February 16, 2021 [Internet]. 2021. Available from: https://www.nccn.org/professionals/physician_gls/pdf/mpm.pdf [Accessed: November 01, 2021]

[2] Bueno R, Stawiski EW, Goldstein LD. Comprehensive genomic analysis of malignant pleural mesothelioma identifies recurrent mutations, gene fusions and splicing alterations. Nature Genetics. 2016;**48**:407-416. DOI: 0.1038/ng.3520

[3] Yap TA, Aerts JG, Popat S. Novel insights into mesothelioma biology and implications for therapy. Nature Reviews Cancer. 2017;**17**:475-488. DOI: 10.1038/nrc.2017.42

[4] Scherpereel A, Wallyn F, Albelda S. Novel medical therapies for malignant pleural mesothelioma: A review. The Lancet Oncology. 2018;**19**:e161-e172. DOI: 10.1016/S1470-2045(18)30100-1

[5] Woolhouse I, Bishop L, Darlison L. British Thoracic Society Guideline for the investigation and management of malignant pleural mesothelioma. Thorax. 2018;**73**(Suppl.1):i1-i30. DOI: 10.1136/thoraxjnl-2017-211321

[6] Kindler HL, Ismaila N, Armato SG 3rd. Treatment of malignant pleural mesothelioma: American Society of Clinical Oncology clinical practice guideline. Journal of Clinical Oncology. 2018;**36**:1343-1373. DOI: 10.1200/JCO.2017.76.6394

[7] Baas P, Fennell D, Kerr KM. Malignant pleural mesothelioma: ESMO Clinical Practice Guidelines for diagnosis, treatment and follow-up. Annals of Oncology. 2015;**26**(Suppl. 5): v31-v39. DOI: 10.1093/annonc/mdv199

[8] Scherpereel A, Opitz I, Berghmans T. ERS/ESTS/EACTS/ESTRO guidelines for the management of malignant pleural mesothelioma. The European Respiratory Journal. 2020;**55**:1900953. DOI: 10.1183/13993003.00953-2019

[9] Sugarbaker DJ. Macroscopic complete resection: The goal of primary surgery in multimodality therapy for pleural mesothelioma. Journal of Thoracic Oncology. 2006;**1**:175-176. DOI: 10.1016/S1556-0864(15)31536-7

[10] Treasure T. What is the best approach for surgery of malignant pleural mesothelioma? It is to put our efforts into obtaining trustworthy evidence for practice. The Journal of Thoracic and Cardiovascular Surgery. 2016;**151**:307-309. DOI: 10.1016/j.jtcvs.2015.09.086

[11] Rusch V, Baldini EH, Bueono R. The role of cytoreduction in the treatment of malignant pleural mesothelioma: Meeting summary of the International Mesothelioma Interest Group Congress, September 11–14, 2012, Boston, MA. Journal of Thoracic Cardiovascular Surgery. 2013;**145**:909-910. DOI: 10.1016/j.jtcvs.2013.01.039

[12] Sugarbaker DJ, Flores RM, Jaklitsch MT. Resection margins, extrapleural nodal status and cell type determine post-operative long term survival in trimodality therapy of malignant pleural mesothelioma: Results in 183 patients. The Journal of Thoracic and Cardiovascular Surgery. 1999;**117**:54-63. DOI: 10.1016/s0022-5223(99)70469-1

[13] Marulli G, Faccioli E, Bellini A. Induction chemotherapy vs post-

operative adjuvant therapy for malignant pleural mesothelioma. Expert Review of Respiratory Medicine. 2017; **11**(8):649-660. DOI: 10.1080/17476348.2017.1338951

[14] Shohdy K, Abdel-Rahman O. The timing of chemotherapy in the management plan for medically operable early-stage malignant pleural mesothelioma. Expert Review of Respiratory Medicine. 2019;**13**(6): 579-584. DOI: 10.1080/17476348.2019.1607300

[15] Burt MB, Lee HS, Raghuram AC. Preoperative prediction of unresectability in malignant pleural mesothelioma. The Journal of Thoracic and Cardiovascular Surgery. 2020;**159**: 2512-2520. DOI: 10.1016/j.jtcvs.2019.11.035

[16] Marulli G, Breda C, Fontana P. Pleurectomy-decortication in malignant pleural mesothelioma: Are different surgical techniques associated with different outcomes? Results from a multicentre study. European Journal of Cardio-Thoracic Surgery. 2017;**52**:63-69. DOI: 10.1093/ejcts/ezx079

[17] Rusch VW, Giroux D, Kennedy C. Initial analysis of the international association for the study of lung cancer mesothelioma database. Journal of Thoracic Oncology. 2012;7:1631-1639. DOI: 10.1097/JTO.0b013e31826915f1

[18] Lang-Lazdunski L, Bille A, Papa S. Pleurectomy/decortication, hyperthermic pleural lavage with povidone-iodine, prophylactic radiotherapy and systemic chemotherapy in patients with malignant pleural mesothelioma: A 10-year experience. The Journal of Thoracic and Cardiovascular Surgery. 2015;**149**: 558-566. DOI: 10.1016/j.jtcvs.2014.10.041

[19] Giles AE, Kidane B. Commentary: Know your enemy–understanding futility in the battle against malignant pleural mesothelioma. The Journal of Thoracic and Cardiovascular Surgery. 2020;**159**:2523-2524. DOI: 10.1016/j.jtcvs.2020.01.034

[20] Bellini A, Dell'Amore A, Giraudo C. Computed tomography and spirometry can predict unresectability in malignant pleural mesothelioma. Journal of Clinical Medicine. 2021;**10**:4407. DOI: 10.3390/jcm10194407

[21] Marulli G, Rea F, Nicotra S. Effect of induction chemotherapy on lung function and exercise capacity in patients affected by malignant pleural mesothelioma. European Journal of Cardio-Thoracic Surgery. 2010;**37**: 1464-1469. DOI: 10.1016/j.ejcts.2010.01.008

[22] Marulli G, Di Chiara F, Braccioni F. Changes in pulmonary function tests predict radiological response to chemotherapy in malignant pleural mesothelioma. European Journal of Cardio-Thoracic Surgery. 2013;**44**: 104-110. DOI: 10.1093/ejcts/ezs624

[23] Sensakovic WF, Armato SG III, Straus C. Computerized segmentation and measurement of malignant pleural mesothelioma. Medical Physics. 2011;**38**: 238-244. DOI: 10.1118/1.3525836

[24] Armato SG III, Nowak AK. Revised modified RECIST criteria for the assessment of response in malignant pleural mesothelioma (version 1.1). Journal of Thoracic Oncology. 2018;**13**: 1012-1021. DOI: 10.1016/j.jtho.2018.04.034

[25] Armato SG III, Sensakovic WF. Automated lung segmentation for thoracic CT: Impact on computer-aided diagnosis. Academic Radiology. 2004;**11**:

1011-1021. DOI: 10.1016/j.acra.2004.06.005

[26] Labby EZ, Armato SG III, Dignam JJ. Lung volume measurements as surrogate marker for patient response in malingant pleural mesothelioma. Journal of Thoracic Oncology. 2013;**8**:478-486. DOI: 10.1097/JTO.0b013e31828354c8

[27] Hashimoto M, Takeuchi J, Teruhisa T. Pleural thickness after neoadjuvant chemotherapy is a prognostic factor in malignant pleural mesothelioma. The Journal of Thoracic and Cardiovascular Surgery. 2019;**157**:404-413. DOI: 10.1016/j.jtcvs.2018.09.106

[28] De Perrot M. Commentary: Is thoracic cage volume a newparameter for clinical staging inmesothelioma? The Journal of Thoracic and Cardiovascular Surgery. 2020;**159**:2520-2521. DOI: 10.1016/j.jtcvs.2019.12.048

[29] Nowak AK, Chansky K, Rice DC. The IASLC Mesothelioma Staging Project: Proposals for revisions of the T descriptors in the forthcoming eighth editions of the TNM classification for mesothelioma. Journal of Thoracic Oncology. 2016;**11**:2089-2099. DOI: 10.1016/j.jtho.2016.08.147

[30] Waller DA, Opitz I, Bueno R. Divided by an ocean of water but united in an ocean of uncertainty: A transatlantic review of mesothelioma surgery guidelines. The Journal of Thoracic and Cardiovascular Surgery. 2021;**161**:1922-1925. DOI: 10.1093/ejcts/ezaa363

[31] Kim S, Bull DA, Garland L. Is there a role for cancer-directed surgery in early-stage sarcomatoid or biphasic mesothelioma? The Annals of Thoracic Surgery. 2019;**107**:194-201. DOI: 10.1016/j.athoracsur.2018.07.081

[32] Lococo F, Torricelli F, Lang-Lazdunski L. Survival results in biphasic malignant pleural mesothelioma patients: A multicentric analysis. The Journal of Thoracic and Cardiovascular Surgery. 2020;**159**(4):1584-1593. DOI: 10.1016/j.jtcvs.2019.08.027

[33] Harling L, Kolokotroni SM, Nair A. Differential survival characteristics of sarcomatoid subtype in biphasic pleural mesothelioma. The Annals of Thoracic Surgery. 2019;**107**(3):929-935. DOI: 10.1016/j.athoracsur.2018.09.019

[34] Rice D, Chansky K, Nowak A. The IASLC Mesothelioma Staging Project: Proposals for revisions of the N descriptors in the forthcoming eighth edition of the TNM classification for pleural mesothelioma. Journal of Thoracic Oncology. 2016;**11**:2100-2111. DOI: 10.1016/j.jtho.2016.09.121

[35] Sugarbaker DJ, Jaklitsch MT, Bueno R. Prevention, early detection, and management of complications after 328 consecutive extrapleural pneumonectomies. The Journal of Thoracic and Cardiovascular Surgery. 2004;**128**:138-146. DOI: 10.1016/j.jtcvs.2004.02.021

[36] Martini N, Bains MS, Beattie EJ Jr. Indications for pleurectomy in malignant effusion. Cancer. 1975;**35**:734-738. DOI: 10.1002/1097-0142(197503)35:3<734::aid-cncr2820350328>3.0.co;2-n

[37] Cao C, Tian DH, Pataky KA. Systematic review of pleurectomy in the treatment of malignant pleural mesothelioma. Lung Cancer. 2013;**81**:39-27. DOI: 10.1016/j.lungcan.2013.04.024

[38] Rice D, Rusch V, Pass H. Recommendation for uniform definitions of surgical techniques for malignant pleural mesothelioma. A

consensus report of the International Association for the Study of Lung Cancer International Staging Committee and the International Mesothelioma Interest Group. Journal of Thoracic Oncology. 2011;**6**:1304-1312. DOI: 10.1097/JTO.0b013e3182208e3f

[39] Bertoglio P, Garelli E, Brandolini J. Surgical management and reconstruction of diaphragm, pericardium and chest wall in mesothelioma surgery: A review. Journal of Clinical Medicine. 2021;**10**:2330. DOI: 10.3390/jcm10112330

[40] Butchart EG, Ashcroft T, Barnsley WC. Pleuropneumonectomy in the management of diffuse pleural mesothelioma of the pleura. Experience with 29 patients. Thorax. 1976;**31**:15-24. DOI: 10.1136/thx.31.1.15

[41] Weder W, Stahel RA, Bernhard J. Multicenter trial of neoadjuvant chemotherapy followed by extrapleural pneumonectomy in malignant pleural mesothelioma. Annals of Oncology. 2007;**18**:1196-1202. DOI: 10.1093/annonc/mdm093

[42] Treasure T, Internullo E, Fiorentino F. A survey of opinions and beliefs concerning surgery for malignant pleural mesothelioma amongst 802 members of the European Association for Cardio Thoracic Surgery (EACTS), the European Society of Thoracic Surgeons (ESTS) and the society of Thoracic Surgeons (STS). Interactive Cardiovascular and Thoracic Surgery. 2011;**12**:341-346. DOI: 10.1510/icvts.2010.251488

[43] Cho BC, Donahoe L, Bradbury PD. Surgery for malignant pleural mesothelioma after radiotherapy (SMART): Final results from a single-centre, phase 2 trial. The Lancet Oncology. 2021;**22**:190-197. DOI: 10.1016/S1470-2045(20)30606-9

[44] Treasure T, Lang-lazdunski L, Waller D. Extrapleural pneumonectomy versus no extrapleural pneumonectomy for patients with malignant pleural mesothelioma: Clinical outcomes of the Mesothelioma and Radical Surgery (MARS) randomized feasibility study. The Lancet Oncology. 2011;**12**:763-772. DOI: 10.1016/S1470-2045(11)70149-8

[45] Weder W, Stahel RA, Baas P. The MARS feasibility trial: Conclusions not supported by data. The Lancet Oncology. 2011;**12**:1093-1094. DOI: 10.1016/S1470-2045(11)70307-2

[46] Wanebo HJ, Martini N, Melamed MR. Pleural mesothelioma. Cancer. 1976;**38**:2481-2488. DOI: 10.1002/1097-0142(197612)38:6<2481::aid-cncr2820380637>3.0.co;2-9

[47] Teh E, Fiorentino F, Tan C. A systematic review of lung sparing extirpative surgery for pleural mesothelioma. Journal of the Royal Society of Medicine. 2011;**104**:69-80. DOI: 10.1258/jrsm.2010.100345

[48] Lim E, Darlison L, Edwards J. Mesothelioma and Radical Surgery 2 (MARS 2): Protocol for a multicentre randomised trial comparing (extended) pleurectomy decortication versus no (extended) pleurectomy decortication for patients with malignant pleural mesothelioma. BMJ Open. 2020;**10**:e038892

[49] Friedberg JS, Culligan MJ, Mick R. Radical pleurectomy and intraoperative photodynamic therapy for malignant pleural mesothelioma. The Annals of Thoracic Surgery. 2012;**93**:1658-1667. DOI: 10.1016/j.athoracsur.2012.02.009

[50] Flores RM. The mesothelioma surgery shift. The Journal of Thoracic and Cardiovascular Surgery. 2016;**151**:

485-486. DOI: 10.1016/j.jtcvs.2015.10.054

[51] Flores RM, Pass HI, Seshan VE. Extrapleural pneumonectomy versus pleurectomy/decortication in the surgical management of malignant pleural mesothelioma results in 663 patients. The Journal of Thoracic and Cardiovascular Surgery. 2008;**135**: 620-626. DOI: 10.1016/j.jtcvs.2007.10.054

[52] Faccioli E, Bellini A, Mammana M. Extrapleural pneumonectomies for pleural mesothelioma. Expert Review of Respiratory Medicine. 2020;**14**(1):67-79. DOI: 10.1080/17476348.2020.1688147

[53] Reeb J, Olland A, Massard G. Extracorporeal life support in thoracic surgery. European Journal of Cardio-Thoracic Surgery. 2018;**53**(03):489-494. DOI: 10.1093/ejcts/ezx477

[54] Extracorporeal Life Support Organization. ELSO Guidelines for Cardiopulmonary Extracorporeal Life Support, Version 1.4, August 2017 Ann Arbor, MI, USA [Internet]. 2017. Available from: https://www.elso.org [Accessed: November 1, 2021]

[55] Tathineni P, Pandya M, Chaar B. The utility of ECMO in patients with hematologic malignancies: A literature review. Cureus. 2020;**12**:e9118. DOI: 10.7759/cureus.9118

[56] Dünser M, HasibederW RM. Successful therapy of severe pneumonia-associated ARDS after pneumonectomy with ECMO and steroids. The Annals of Thoracic Surgery. 2004;**78**(01):335-337. DOI: 10.1016/S0003-4975(03)01264-5

[57] Fica M, Suarez F, Aparicio R. Single site venovenous ECMO as an alternative to invasive ventilation in post-pneumonectomy fistula with acute respiratory failure. European Journal of Cardio-Thoracic Surgery. 2012;**41**: 950-952. DOI: 10.1093/ejcts/ezr103

[58] Hadem J, Schroder F, Winkler T. One day from dyspnea to death: Unsuccessful application of ECMO in toxoplasma myocarditis following bone marrow transplantation. Clinical Research in Cardiology. 2006;**95**:477-481. DOI: 10.1007/s00392-006-0402-y

[59] Burt BM, Cameron RB, Mollberg NM. Malignant pleural mesothelioma and the Society of Thoracic Surgeons Database: An analysis of surgical morbidity and mortality. The Journal of Thoracic and Cardiovascular Surgery. 2014;**148**(01):30-35. DOI: 10.1016/j.jtcvs.2014.03.011

[60] Bellini A, Dell'Amore A, Ferrigno P. ECLS for life-threatening complications in mesothelioma's surgery: Is it worthwhile? The Thoracic and Cardiovascular Surgeon. 2021;**69**(6): 548-550. DOI: 10.1055/s-0041-1724037

[61] Gow KW, Lao OB, Leong T. Extracorporeal life support for adults with malignancy and respiratory or cardiac failure: The Extracorporeal Life Support experience. American Journal of Surgery. 2010;**199**(05):669-675. DOI: 10.1016/j.amjsurg.2010.01.018

[62] Rintoul RC, Ritchie AJ, Edwards JG. Efficacy and cost of video-assisted thoracoscopic partial pleurectomy versus talc pleurodesis in patients with malignant pleural mesothelioma (MesoVATS): An open-label, randomised, controlled trial. Lancet. 2014;**384**:1118-1127. DOI: 10.1016/S0140-6736(14)60418-9

[63] Kostron A, Friess M, Crameri O. Relapse pattern and second-line treatment following multimodality treatment for malignant pleural

mesothelioma. European Journal of Cardio-Thoracic Surgery. 2016;**49**: 1516-1523. DOI: 10.1093/ejcts/ezv398

[64] Takuwa T, Hashimoto M, Matsumoto S. Post-recurrence chemotherapy for mesothelioma patients undergoing extrapleural pneumonectomy. International Journal of Clinical Oncology. 2017;**22**:857-864. DOI: 10.1007/s10147-017-1126-x

[65] Kai Y, Tsutani Y, Tsubokawa N. Prolonged post-recurrence survival following pleurectomy/decortication for malignant pleural mesothelioma. Oncology Letters. 2019;**17**:3607-3614. DOI: 10.3892/ol.2019.9979

[66] Soldera SV, Kavanagh J, Pintilie M. Systemic therapy use and outcomes after relapse from preoperative radiation and extrapleural pneumonectomy for malignant pleural mesothelioma. The Oncologist. 2019;**24**:e510-e517. DOI: 10.1634/theoncologist.2018-0501

[67] Nakamura A, Takuwa T, Hashimoto M. Clinical outcomes with recurrence after pleurectomy/ decortication for malignant pleural mesothelioma. The Annals of Thoracic Surgery. 2020;**109**:1537-1543. DOI: 10.1016/j.athoracsur.2019.11.048

[68] Politi L, Borzellino G. Second surgery for recurrence of malignant pleural mesothelioma after extrapleural pneumonectomy. The Annals of Thoracic Surgery. 2010;**89**:207-211. DOI: 10.1016/j.athoracsur.2009.09.028

[69] Okamoto T, Yano T, Haro A. Treatment for recurrence after extrapleural pneumonectomy for malignant pleural mesothelioma: A single institution experience. Thorac Cancer. 2013;**4**(1):66-70. DOI: 10.1111/ j.1759-7714.2012.00138.x

[70] Burt BM, Ali SO, DaSilva MC. Clinical indications and results after chest wall resection for recurrent mesothelioma. The Journal of Thoracic and Cardiovascular Surgery. 2013; **146**(6):1373-1379. DOI: 10.1016/j. jtcvs.2013.07.012

[71] Bellini A, Dell'Amore A, Terzi S. Relapse patterns and tailored treatments strategies for malignant pleural mesothelioma recurrence after multimodality therapy. Journal of Clinical Medicine. 2021;**10**(5):1134. DOI: 10.3390/jcm10051134

[72] Baldini EH, Recht A, Strauss GM. Patterns of failure after trimodality therapy for malignant pleural mesothelioma. The Annals of Thoracic Surgery. 1997;**63**:334-338. DOI: 10.1016/ s0003-4975(96)01228-3

[73] Elsayed HH, Hassaballa AS, Ahmed TA. Recurrence of mesothelioma after a macroscopic complete resection procedure: Is a second radical surgery justified? Interactive Cardiovascular and Thoracic Surgery. 2021;**32**:761-763. DOI: 10.1093/icvts/ivaa338

[74] Cao C, Tian D, Park J. A systematic review and meta-analysis of surgical treatments for malignant pleural mesothelioma. Lung Cancer. 2014;**83**: 240-245. DOI: 10.1016/j.lungcan.2013. 11.026

[75] Van Schil PE, Opitz I, Weder W. Multimodal management of malignant pleural mesothelioma: Where are we today? The European Respiratory Journal. Sep 2014;**44**(3):754-764. DOI: 10.1183/09031936.00207213

[76] Lee DS, Carollo A, Alpert N. VATS pleurectomy decortication is a reasonable alternative for higher risk patients in the management of malignant pleural mesothelioma: An analysis of

short-term outcomes. Cancers (Basel). 2021;**13**(5):1068. DOI: 10.3390/cancers13051068

[77] Opitz I, Weder W. Pleural mesothelioma: Is the surgeon still there? Annals of Oncology. 2018;**29**(8): 1710-1717. DOI: 10.1093/annonc/mdy195

[78] Nelson DB, Rice DC, Mitchell KG. Defining the role of adjuvant radiotherapy for malignant pleural mesothelioma: A propensity-matched landmark analysis of the National Cancer Database. Journal of Thoracic Disease. 2019;**11**(4):1269-1278. DOI: 10.21037/jtd.2019.04.27

[79] Spaggiari L, Marulli G, Bovolato P. Extrapleural pneumonectomy for malignant mesothelioma: An Italian multicenter retrospective study. The Annals of Thoracic Surgery. 2014;**97**: 1859-1865. DOI: 10.1016/j.athoracsur.2014.01.050

[80] Sugarbaker DJ, Wolf AS. Surgery for malignant pleural mesothelioma. Expert Review of Respiratory Medicine. 2010;**4**: 363-372. DOI: 10.1586/ers.10.35

[81] Flores RM. Pleurectomy decortication for mesothelioma: The procedure of choice when possible. The Journal of Thoracic and Cardiovascular Surgery. 2016;**151**:310-312. DOI: 10.1016/j.jtcvs.2015.10.036

[82] Lang-Lazdunski L, Bille A, Lal R. Pleurectomy/decortication is superior to extrapleural pneumonectomy in the multimodality management of patients with malignant pleural mesothelioma. Journal of Thoracic Oncology. 2012;7: 737-743. DOI: 10.1097/JTO.0b013e31824ab6c5

[83] Batirel HF, Metintas M, Caglar HB. Adoption of pleurectomy and decortication for malignant mesothelioma leads to similar survival as extrapleural pneumonectomy. The Journal of Thoracic and Cardiovascular Surgery. 2016;**151**:478-484. DOI: 10.1016/j.jtcvs.2015.09.121

[84] Rena O, Casadio C. Extrapleural pneumonectomy for early stage malignant pleural mesothelioma: A harmful procedure. Lung Cancer. 2012; **77**:151-155. DOI: 10.1016/j.lungcan.2011.12.009

[85] Magouliotis DE, Tasiopoulou VS, Athanassiadi K. Updated meta-analysis of survival after extrapleural pneumonectomy versus pleurectomy/decortication in mesothelioma. General Thoracic and Cardiovascular Surgery. 2019;**67**:312-320. DOI: 10.1007/s11748-018-1027-6

[86] Vigneswaran WT, Kircheva DY, Rodrigues AE. Influence of pleurectomy and decortication in health-related quality of life among patients with malignant pleural mesothelioma. World Journal of Surgery. 2018;**42**:1036-1045. DOI: 10.1007/s00268-017-4264-4

[87] Papaspyros S. Surgical management of malignant pleural mesothelioma: Impact of surgery on survival and quality of life—relation to chemotherapy, radiotherapy, and alternative therapies. ISRN Surgery. 2014;**2014**:817203. DOI: 10.1155/2014/817203

[88] Kostron A, Friess M, Inci I. Propensity matched comparison of extrapleural pneumonectomy and pleurectomy/decortication for mesothelioma patients. Interactive Cardiovascular and Thoracic Surgery. 2017;**24**:740-746. DOI: 10.1093/icvts/ivw422

[89] Sharkey AJ, Tenconi S. Nakas A The effects of an intentional transition from

extrapleural pneumonectomy to extended pleurectomy/decortication. European Journal of Cardio-Thoracic Surgery. 2016;**49**:1632-1641. DOI: 10.1093/ejcts/ezv403

[90] Bueno R, Opitz I, IASCL Mesothelioma Taskforce. Surgery in malignant pleural mesothelioma. Journal of Thoracic Oncology. 2018;**13**: 1638-1654. DOI: 10.1016/j.jtho.2018.08.001

[91] Datta A, Smith R, Fiorentino F. Surgery in the treatment of malignant pleural mesothelioma: Recruitment into trials should be the default position. Thorax. 2014;**69**:194-197. DOI: 10.1136/thoraxjnl-2013-203846

[92] Treasure T, Sedrakyan A. Pleural mesothelioma: Little evidence, still time to do trials. Lancet. 2004;**364**:1183-1185. DOI: 10.1016/S0140-6736(04)17108-0

[93] Fournel L, Janet-Vendroux A, Canny-Hamelin E. Malignant pleural mesothelioma: The role of surgery. Revue de Pneumologie Clinique. 2018; **74**:351-358. DOI: 10.1016/j.pneumo.2018.09.006

[94] Treasure T, Macbeth F. Fifteen years in the evaluation of extrapleural pneumonectomy: Lessons to be learned. The Journal of Thoracic and Cardiovascular Surgery. 2015;**149**: 1382-1383. DOI: 10.1016/j.jtcvs.2014.10.083

[95] Hiddinga BI, van Meerbeeck JP. Surgery in mesothelioma-where do we go after MARS? Journal of Thoracic Oncology. 2013;**8**:525-529. DOI: 10.1097/JTO.0b013e31828353d7

[96] van Zandwijk N, Clarke C, Henderson D. Guidelines for the diagnosis and treatment of malignant pleural mesothelioma. Journal of Thoracic Disease. 2013;**5**:E254. DOI: 10.3978/j.issn.2072-1439.2013.11.28

[97] Scherpereel A, Astoul P, Baas P. Guidelines of the European Respiratory Society and the European Society of Thoracic Surgeons for the management of malignant pleural mesothelioma. The European Respiratory Journal. 2010;**35**: 479-495. DOI: 10.1183/09031936.00063109

[98] Fahrner R, Ochsenbein A, Schmid RA. Long term survival after trimodal therapy in malignant pleural mesothelioma. Swiss Medical Weekly. 2012;**142**:w13686. DOI: 10.4414/smw.2012.13686

[99] Ceresoli GL, Castagneto B, Zucali PA. Pemetrexed plus carboplatin in elderly patients with malignant pleural mesothelioma: Combined analysis of two phase II trials. British Journal of Cancer. 2008;**99**:51-56. DOI: 10.1038/sj.bjc.6604442

[100] Katirtzoglou N, Gkiozos I, Makrilia N. Carboplatin plus pemetrexed as first-line treatment of patients with malignant pleural mesothelioma: A Phase II Study. Clinical Lung Cancer. 2010;**11**:30-35. DOI: 10.3816/CLC.2010.n.005

[101] Ceresoli GL, Zucali PA, Favaretto AG. Phase II Study of pemetrexed plus carboplatin in malignant pleural mesothelioma. Journal of Clinical Oncology. 2006;**24**: 1443-1448. DOI: 10.1200/JCO.2005.04.3190

[102] Zalcman G, Mazieres J, Margery J. Bevacizumab for newly diagnosed pleural mesothelioma in the Mesothelioma Avastin Cisplatin Pemetrexed Study (MAPS): A randomised, controlled, open-label, phase 3 trial. Lancet. 2016;**387**:

1405-1414. DOI: 10.1016/S0140-6736 (15)01238-6

[103] Jassem J, Ramlau R, Santoro A. Phase III trial of pemetrexed plus best supportive care compared with best supportive care in previously treated patients with advanced malignant pleural mesothelioma. Journal of Clinical Oncology. 2008;**26**:1698-1704. DOI: 10.1200/JCO.2006.09.9887

[104] Muers MF, Stephens RJ, Fisher P. Active symptom control with or without chemotherapy in the treatment of patients with malignant pleural mesothelioma (MS01): A multicentre randomised trial. Lancet. 2008;**371**: 1685-1694. DOI: 10.1016/S0140-6736 (08)60727-8

[105] Richards WG, Zellos L, Bueno R. Phase I to II study of pleurectomy/ decortication and intraoperative intracavitary hyperthermic cisplatin lavage for mesothelioma. Journal of Clinical Oncology. 2006;**24**:1561-1567. DOI: 10.1200/JCO.2005.04.6813

[106] Gomez D, Tsao AS. Local and systemic therapies for malignant pleural mesothelioma. Current Treatment Options in Oncology. 2014;**15**:683-699. DOI: 10.1007/s11864-014-0314-4

[107] Burt BM, Richards WG, Lee HS. A Phase I Trial of surgical resection and intraoperative hyperthermic cisplatin and gemcitabine for pleural mesothelioma. Journal of Thoracic Oncology. 2018;**13**:1400-1409. DOI: 10.1016/j.jtho.2018.04.032

[108] Bertoglio P, Aprile V, Ambrogi MC. The role of intracavitary therapies in the treatment of malignant pleural mesothelioma. Journal of Thoracic Disease. 2018;**10**:S293-S297. DOI: 10.21037/jtd.2017.10.165

[109] Opitz I, Lauk O, Meerang M. Intracavitary cisplatin-fibrin chemotherapy after surgery for malignant pleural mesothelioma: A phase I trial. The Journal of Thoracic and Cardiovascular Surgery. 2020;**159**: 330-340. DOI: 10.1016/j. jtcvs.2019.07.073

[110] Okabe K. Intraoperative intracavitary hyperthermic chemotherapy for malignant pleural mesothelioma. Annals of Translational Medicine. 2017;**5**:233. DOI: 10.21037/ atm.2017.03.78

[111] Ried M, Potzger T, Braune N. Local and systemic exposure of cisplatin during hyperthermic intrathoracic chemotherapy perfusion after pleurectomy and decortication for treatment of pleural malignancies. Journal of Surgical Oncology. 2013;**107**: 735-740. DOI: 10.1002/jso.23321

[112] Ishibashi H, Kobayashi M, Takasaki C. Interim results of pleurectomy/decortication and intraoperative intrapleural hyperthermic cisplatin perfusion for patients with malignant pleural mesothelioma intolerable to extrapleural pneumonectomy. General Thoracic and Cardiovascular Surgery. 2015;**63**: 395-400. DOI: 10.1007/s11748-015-0535-x

[113] Sugarbaker DJ, Gill RR, Yeap BY. Hyperthermic intraoperative pleural cisplatin chemotherapy extends interval to recurrence and survival among low-risk patients with malignant pleural mesothelioma undergoing surgical macroscopic complete resection. The Journal of Thoracic and Cardiovascular Surgery. 2013;**145**:955-963. DOI: 10.1016/j.jtcvs.2012.12.037

[114] Rusch VW, Rosenzweig K, Venkatraman E. A phase II trial of

surgical resection and adjuvant high-dose hemithoracic radiation for malignant pleural mesothelioma. The Journal of Thoracic and Cardiovascular Surgery. 2001;**122**:788-795. DOI: 10.1067/mtc.2001.116560

[115] Buduhan G, Menon S, Aye R. Trimodality therapy for malignant pleural mesothelioma. The Annals of Thoracic Surgery. 2009;**88**:870-875. DOI: 10.1016/j.athoracsur.2009.05.036

[116] de Perrot M, Feld R, Cho BC. Trimodality therapy with induction chemotherapy followed by extrapleural pneumonectomy and adjuvant high-dose hemithoracic radiation for malignant pleural mesothelioma. Journal of Clinical Oncology. 2009;**27**:1413-1418. DOI: 10.1200/JCO.2008.17.5604

[117] Kapeles M, Gensheimer MF, Mart DA. Trimodality treatment of malignant pleural mesothelioma: An institutional review. American Journal of Clinical Oncology. 2018;**41**:30-35. DOI: 10.1097/COC.0000000000000225

[118] Thieke C, Nicolay NH, Sterzing F. Long-term results in malignant pleural mesothelioma treated with neoadjuvant chemotherapy, extrapleural pneumonectomy and intensity-modulated radiotherapy. Radiation Oncology. 2015;**10**:267. DOI: 10.1186/s13014-015-0575-5

[119] Mencoboni M, Filiberti RA, Taveggia P. Clinical features and treatment outcome of malignant pleural mesothelioma. Oncology Research and Treatment. 2017;**40**:364-369. DOI: 10.1159/000464410

[120] Rea F, Marulli G, Bortolotti L. Induction chemotherapy, extrapleural pneumonectomy (EPP) and adjuvant hemi-thoracic radiation in malignant pleural mesothelioma (MPM): Feasibility and results. Lung Cancer. 2007;**57**:89-95. DOI: 10.1016/j.lungcan.2007.02.004

[121] Van Schil PE, Baas P, Gaafar R. Trimodality therapy for malignant pleural mesothelioma: Results from an EORTC phase II multicentre trial. The European Respiratory Journal. 2010;**36**:1362-1369. DOI: 10.1183/09031936.00039510

[122] Krug LM, Pass HI, Rusch VW. Multicenter phase II trial of neoadjuvant pemetrexed plus cisplatin followed by extrapleural pneumonectomy and radiation for malignant pleural mesothelioma. Journal of Clinical Oncology. 2009;**27**:3007-2013. DOI: 10.1200/JCO.2008.20.3943

[123] Gomez DR, Rimner A, Simone CB 2nd. The use of radiation therapy for the treatment of malignant pleural mesothelioma: Expert Opinion from the National Cancer Institute Thoracic Malignancy Steering Committee, International Association for the Study of Lung Cancer, and Mesothelioma Applied Research Foundation. Journal of Thoracic Oncology. 2019;**14**:1172-1183. DOI: 10.1016/j.jtho.2019.03.030

[124] Rice DC, Stevens CW, Correa AM. Outcomes after extrapleural pneumonectomy and intensity-modulated radiation therapy for malignant pleural mesothelioma. The Annals of Thoracic Surgery. 2007;**84**:1685-1692. DOI: 10.1016/j.athoracsur.2007.04.076

[125] Gomez DR, Hong DS, Allen PK. Patterns of failure, toxicity, and survival after extrapleural pneumonectomy and hemithoracic intensity-modulated radiation therapy for malignant pleural mesothelioma. Journal of Thoracic Oncology. 2013;**8**:238-245. DOI: 10.1097/JTO.0b013e31827740f0

[126] Rimner A, Zauderer MG, Gomez DR. Phase II study of hemithoracic intensity-modulated pleural radiation therapy (IMPRINT) as part of lung-sparing multimodality therapy in patients with malignant pleural mesothelioma. Journal of Clinical Oncology. 2016;**34**:2761. DOI: 10.1200/JCO.2016.67.2675

[127] Shaikh F, Zauderer MG, von Reibnitz D. Improved outcomes with modern lung-sparing trimodality therapy in patients with malignant pleural mesothelioma. Journal of Thoracic Oncology. 2017;**12**:993-1000. DOI: 10.1016/j.jtho.2017.02.026

[128] Espinoza-Mercado F, Borgella JD, Berz D. Disparities in compliance with national guidelines for the treatment of malignant pleural mesothelioma. The Annals of Thoracic Surgery. 2019;**108**: 889-896. DOI: 10.1016/j.athoracsur.2019.03.052

[129] Ahamad A, Stevens CW, Smythe WR. Promising early local control of malignant pleural mesothelioma following postoperative intensity modulated radiotherapy (IMRT) to the chest. Cancer Journal. 2003;**9**:476-484. DOI: 10.1097/00130404-200311000-00008

[130] Vogelzang NJ, Rusthoven JJ, Symanowski J. Phase III study of pemetrexed in combination with cisplatin versus cisplatin alone in patients with malignant pleural mesothelioma. Journal of Clinical Oncology. 2003;**21**:2636-2644. DOI: 10.1200/JCO.2003.11.136

[131] Sandin LC, Eriksson F, Ellmark P. Local CTLA4 blockade effectively restrains experimental pancreatic adenocarcinoma growth in vivo. Oncoimmunology. 2014;**3**:e27614. DOI: 10.4161/onci.27614

[132] Fransen MF, van der Sluis TC, Ossendorp F. Controlled local delivery of CTLA-4 blocking antibody induces CD8+ T-cell-dependent tumor eradication and decreases risk of toxic side effects. Clinical Cancer Research. 2013;**19**:5381-5389. DOI: 10.1158/1078-0432.CCR-12-0781

[133] Popat S, Curioni-Fontecedro A, Polydoropoulou V. A multicentre randomized phase III trial comparing pembrolizumab (P) vs single agent chemotherapy (CT) for advanced pre-treated malignant pleural mesothelioma (MPM): Results from the European Thoracic Oncology Platform (ETOP 9-15) PROMISE-meso trial. Annals of Oncology. 2020;**31**(12):1734-1745. DOI: 10.1016/j.annonc.2020.09.009

[134] Scherpereel A, Mazieres J, Greillier L. Nivolumab or nivolumab plus ipilimumab in patients with relapsed malignant pleural mesothelioma (IFCT-1501 MAPS2): A multicentre, open-label, randomised, non-comparative, phase 2 trial. The Lancet Oncology. 2019;**20**:239-253. DOI: 10.1016/S1470-2045(18)30765-4

[135] Menis J, Pasello G, Remon J. Immunotherapy in malignant pleural mesothelioma: A review of literature data. Transl Lung Cancer Res. 2021; **10**(6):2988-3000. DOI: 10.21037/tlcr-20-673

[136] Baas P, Scherpereel A, Nowak AK. First-line nivolumab plus ipilimumab in unresectable malignant pleural mesothelioma (CheckMate 743): A multicentre, randomised, open-label, phase 3 trial. Lancet. 2021;**397**(10272): 375-386. DOI: 10.1016/S0140-6736(20)32714-8

[137] CheckpOiNt Blockade For Inhibition of Relapsed Mesothelioma (CONFIRM) [Internet]. 2017. Available from: https://www.clinicaltrials.gov/ct2/

show/NCT03063450 [Accessed: November 01, 2021]

[138] Nowak AK, Brosseau S, Cook A. Antiangiogeneic strategies in mesothelioma. Frontier in Oncologia. 2020;**10**:126. DOI: 10.3389/fonc.2020.00126

[139] Aprile G, Rijavec E, Fontanella C. Ramucirumab: Preclinical research and clinical development. Oncotargets and Therapy. 2014;**7**:1997-2006. DOI: 10.2147/OTT.S61132

[140] Désage AL, Karpathiou G, Peoc'h M. The immune microenvironment of malignant pleural mesothelioma: A literature review. Cancers (Basel). 2021; **13**(13):3205. DOI: 10.3390/cancers13133205

[141] Pinto C, Zucali PA, Pagano M. Gemcitabine with or without ramucirumab as second-line treatment for malignant pleural mesothelioma (RAMES): A randomised, double-blind, placebo-controlled, phase 2 trial. The Lancet Oncology. 2021;**22**(10): 1438-1447. DOI: 10.1016/S1470-2045(21)00404-6

[142] Maio M, Scherpereel A, Calabro L. Tremelimumab as second-line or third-line treatment in relapsed malignant mesothelioma (DETERMINE): A multicentre, international, randomised, double-blind, placebo-controlled phase 2b trial. The Lancet Oncology. 2017;**18**: 1261-1273. DOI: 10.1016/S1470-2045(17)30446-1

[143] Adusumilli PS, Zauderer MG, Rusch VW. Regional delivery of mesothelin-targeted CAR T cells for pleural cancers: Safety and preliminary efficacy in combination with anti-PD-1 agent. Journal of Clinical Oncology. 2019;**37**:2511. DOI: 10.1200/JCO.2019.37.15_suppl.2511

[144] Chong EA, Svoboda J, Dwivedy NS. Sequential anti-CD19 directed chimeric antigen receptor modified T-cell therapy (CART19) and PD-1 blockade with pembrolizumab in patients with relapsed or refractory B-cell non-Hodgkin Lymphomas. Blood. 2018;**132**:4198. DOI: 10.3389/fonc.2019.00767

[145] Zauderer MG, Tsao AS, Dao T. A Randomized Phase II Trial of Adjuvant Galinpepimut-S, WT-1 analogue peptide vaccine, after multimodality therapy for patients with malignant pleural mesothelioma. Clinical Cancer Research. 2017;**23**:7483-7489. DOI: 10.1158/1078-0432.CCR-17-2169

[146] Gabrilovich DI, Ciernik IF, Carbone DP. Dendritic cells in antitumor immune responses. I. Defective antigen presentation in tumor-bearing hosts. Cellular Immunology. 1996;**170**:101-110. DOI: 10.1006/cimm.1996.0139

[147] Enk AH, Jonuleit H, Saloga J. Dendritic cells as mediators of tumor-induced tolerance in metastatic melanoma. International Journal of Cancer. 1997;**73**:309-316. DOI: 10.1002/(sici)1097-0215(19971104)73:3<309::aid-ijc1>3.0.co;2-3

[148] Muggerud AA, Hallett M, Johnsen H. Molecular diversity in ductal carcinoma in situ (DCIS) and early invasive breast cancer. Molecular Oncology. 2010;**4**:357-368. DOI: 10.1016/j.molonc.2010.06.007

[149] Grosso F, Steele N, Novello S. Nintedanib plus pemetrexed/cisplatin in patients with malignant pleural mesothelioma: Phase II results from the Randomized, Placebo-Controlled LUME-Meso Trial. Journal of Clinical Oncology. 2017;**35**:3591-3600. DOI: 10.1200/JCO.2017.72.9012

[150] Scagliotti GV, Gaafar R, Nowak AK. Nintedanib in combination with pemetrexed and cisplatin for chemotherapy-naive patients with advanced malignant pleural mesothelioma (LUME-Meso): A double-blind, randomised, placebo-controlled phase 3 trial. The Lancet Respiratory Medicine. 2019;**7**:569-580. DOI: 10.1016/S2213-2600(19)30139-0

[151] Kelly WK, O'Connor OA, Krug LM. Phase I study of an oral histone deacetylase inhibitor, suberoylanilide hydroxamic acid, in patients with advanced cancer. Journal of Clinical Oncology. 2005;**23**:3923-3931. DOI: 10.1200/JCO.2005.14.167

[152] Krug LM, Kindler HL, Calvert H. Vorinostat in patients with advanced malignant pleural mesothelioma who have progressed on previous chemotherapy (VANTAGE-014): A phase 3, double-blind, randomised, placebo-controlled trial. The Lancet Oncology. 2015;**16**:447-456. DOI: 10.1016/S1470-2045(15)70056-2

Chapter 6

Recent Advances in Systemic Therapy for Malignant Pleural Mesothelioma: Focus on Anti-Angiogenic Inhibitors and Immune Checkpoint Inhibitors

Fumie Onishi and Nobukazu Fujimoto

Abstract

Malignant pleural mesothelioma (MPM) is a neoplasm strongly associated with past exposure to asbestos. In general, the prognosis of patients with MPM is poor; however, in recent years, some encouraging results have been reported for systemic therapies for MPM. In a randomized phase III study, the combination of nivolumab and ipilimumab improved overall survival, compared to the standard platinum-based chemotherapy. An important clinical issue is whether the outcome of patients with MPM might be further improved by combining immunotherapies with cytotoxic chemotherapy and/or angiogenesis inhibitors. This chapter covers recent findings on systemic therapies, including cytotoxic chemotherapy, anti-angiogenic inhibitors, and/or immune checkpoint inhibitors.

Keywords: anti-angiogenic inhibitors, asbestos, immune checkpoint inhibitors, Ipilimumab, nivolumab

1. Introduction

Malignant pleural mesothelioma (MPM) is a rare neoplasm with a poor prognosis. MPM is strongly associated with past exposure to asbestos [1]. Radical surgeries, such as an extrapleural pneumonectomy or pleural decortication, have been performed for treating patients with MPM previously, but favorable results have been observed in only a limited number of patients [2, 3]. Most patients that present with advanced, non-resectable MPM at diagnosis are candidates for systemic treatments. However, systemic chemotherapy can only be administered to patients with good performance status (PS) [4].

In 2003, Vogelzang et al. reported that the combination of pemetrexed and cisplatin (pemetrexed/cisplatin) improved the response rate (RR), progression-free survival (PFS), and overall survival (OS), compared to cisplatin alone [5]. Since then, systemic chemotherapy with platinum and pemetrexed combination has been considered standard therapy for advanced MPM. However, even with this treatment, the PFS and OS have been estimated at 5.7 months and 12.1 months, respectively [5, 6]. A second-line treatment has not been established. According to the US Surveillance, Epidemiology, and End Results Medicare investigation, the most common second-line treatments are pemetrexed-based retreatment or gemcitabine [6].

There is strong evidence that angiogenesis is an important determinant in the development and progression of MPM. There are two main targets for inhibiting angiogenesis. One is the potent mitogen for endothelial cells, vascular endothelial growth factor (VEGF), which transduces signals by binding to two receptors, VEGF receptors −1 and 2. The other is platelet-derived growth factor (PDGF), which functions as an autocrine growth stimulator in the pathogenesis of MPM [7, 8]. With the introduction of angiogenesis inhibitors, several clinical studies have investigated treatments for MPM.

An alternative approach is to target the complex interaction between cancer and host immunity: cancer cells can acquire the ability to evade the host immune system, which curtails their growth [9, 10]. Cancer cells can also actively subvert the immunosuppressive function of T cells and immune checkpoint molecules, such as cytotoxic T lymphocyte antigen (CTLA)-4, programmed cell death (PD)-1, and PD-ligand (PD-L)-1. In recent years, immune checkpoint inhibitors (ICIs) have shown remarkable results in treating multiple types of neoplasms. The etiology and pathogenesis of MPM are mostly attributed to the generation of an immune microenvironment favorable to tumor growth, caused by asbestos-induced damage [11]. There is evidence that ICIs might play an important role in the treatment of MPM; in fact, some encouraging results have emerged in recent years.

Here, we discuss the results of recent trials on systemic therapies against MPM, with a focus on anti-angiogenic inhibitors and ICIs.

2. Angiogenesis inhibitors

Most early studies on anti-angiogenic agents explored their clinical efficacy as single drugs for treating cancer in the relapsed or recurrent setting. However, the outcome of those studies was generally disappointing. Later, anti-angiogenic agents were combined with cytotoxic agents, mainly pemetrexed/cisplatin.

Bevacizumab is a monoclonal antibody that binds VEGF-A. Bevacizumab was tested in combination with the standard-of-care, cisplatin and pemetrexed, as a first-line treatment. An open-label, randomized phase 2/3 study that added bevacizumab to cisplatin and pemetrexed in chemotherapy-naïve patients showed a beneficial effect [12]. In that study, 448 patients were randomized to either pemetrexed/cisplatin with bevacizumab or chemotherapy alone. Patients were treated for up to 6 cycles. OS was statistically prolonged in the bevacizumab arm; the median OS was 18.8 months, versus 16.1 months for chemotherapy alone (HR: 0.77, 95% CI: 0.62–0.95).

Nintedanib is a multi-target angiokinase inhibitor, with activity against the receptors for VEGF (receptors 1, 2, and 3), PDGF, and fibroblast growth factor. A phase II study on patients with MPM showed that the addition of nintedanib to pemetrexed/cisplatin improved PFS (median 9.4 vs. 5.7 months; hazard ratio [HR]: 0.54; 95% CI: 0.33–0.87; p = 0.010). Moreover, the nintedanib arm showed a trend toward improved OS (median 18.3 vs. 14.2 months; HR: 0.77; 95% CI: 0.46–1.29; p = 0.319), compared to placebo. These positive effects were observed in patients with epithelioid histology. However, the findings were not confirmed in the subsequent phase 3 study [13].

Recently, ramucirumab, an anti-VEGF receptor-2 antibody, was tested in a double-blind, placebo-controlled, phase 2 trial for patients with pretreated MPM. In that trial, 161 patients were randomly assigned to gemcitabine (1000 mg/m^2 intravenously, on days 1 and 8 every 3 weeks) or gemcitabine plus ramucirumab (10 mg/kg, intravenously, on day 1 every 3 weeks) [14]. The OS was prolonged in the ramucirumab arm (HR: 0·71, 70% CI: 0·59–0·85; p = 0·028); the median OS was 13·8 months (70% CI: 12·7–14·4) with gemcitabine plus ramucirumab and 7·5 months (70% CI: 6·9–8·9) with gemcitabine plus placebo. Hypertension was more common in the gemcitabine plus ramucirumab group, but no events were related to bleeding.

3. Immune checkpoint inhibitors

Anti-CTLA-4 antibodies include tremelimumab and ipilimumab. Drugs that block PD-(L)-1 include pembrolizumab, nivolumab, durvalumab, and avelumab.

3.1 Nivolumab monotherapy

The MERIT trial was a phase 2, single-phase study that evaluated the safety and efficacy of nivolumab in Japanese patients with advanced or recurrent MPM, who were refractory or intolerant to 1–2 regimens of therapy [15]. In that study, 34 patients received nivolumab (240 mg intravenously) every 2 weeks, until they displayed progressive disease or unacceptable toxicity. The primary endpoint was the objective RR, which was 29.4% (10/34). The median OS and PFS times were 17.3 and 6.1 months, respectively. Among the 34 patients, 11 (32%) experienced grades ≥3 treatment-related adverse events, including 4 patients (12%) with adverse events that led to study treatment discontinuation (2 events of interstitial pneumonia, and 2 events of pneumonitis). Based on those results, nivolumab was approved for patients with MPM that were refractory or intolerant to prior chemotherapy.

The therapeutic efficacy of nivolumab was confirmed in a phase III trial, which demonstrated that single-agent nivolumab provided a significant improvement in both OS and PFS [16]. In that study, 332 adult patients with previously treated, unresectable, histologically confirmed malignant mesothelioma were randomized to nivolumab or placebo. The median OS was immature, but it was significantly prolonged with nivolumab (9.2 vs. 6.6 months; HR: 0.72; 95% CI: 0.55–0.94; p = 0.02). The median PFS was also prolonged with nivolumab compared to placebo (3.0 vs. 1.8 months; HR: 0.62; 95% CI: 0.49–0.78; p < 0.001). Grades 3–4 treatment-related adverse events occurred in 19% of the nivolumab arm and 6.3% of the placebo arm. Treatment discontinuation due to toxicity occurred in 13.1% of the nivolumab arm, versus 2.7% of the placebo arm.

3.2 ICI-ICI combination

The MAPS2 trial was a multicenter randomized, open-label, phase 2 trial that investigated nivolumab plus ipilimumab versus single-agent nivolumab, as a salvage treatment [17]. In the intention-to-treat population, 12-week disease control was achieved by 32 of 62 patients (52%; 95% CI: 39–64) in the nivolumab plus ipilimumab group and 25 of 63 patients (40%; 95% CI: 28–52) in the nivolumab group. Asthenia was among the most frequent grade 3 adverse events (n = 3 [5%] in the combination arm and n = 1 [2%] in the nivolumab arm).

The CheckMate 743 trial was a global, open-label, randomized, phase 3 study that investigated first-line nivolumab plus ipilimumab versus the standard platinum plus pemetrexed chemotherapy [18]. In that study, 605 patients with previously untreated, unresectable MPM were randomly assigned to nivolumab (3 mg/kg intravenously once every 2 weeks) plus ipilimumab (1 mg/kg intravenously once every 6 weeks), administered for up to 2 years, or platinum (cisplatin or carboplatin) plus pemetrexed chemotherapy, administered once every 3 weeks for up to 6 cycles. The primary endpoint was OS. The OS was significantly extended in the nivolumab plus ipilimumab arm, with a median of 18.1 months (95% CI: 16.8–21.4), compared to 14.1 months (95% CI: 12.4–16.2) in the chemotherapy arm. The HR was 0.74 (96.6% CI: 0.60–0.91). The 1-year and 2-year OS rates were, respectively, 68% (95% CI: 62.3–72.8) and 41% (95% CI: 35.1–46.5) in the nivolumab plus ipilimumab arm, and 58% (95% CI: 51.7–63.2) and 27% (95% CI: 21.9–32.4) in the chemotherapy arm. Across most subgroups, OS was more favorable with nivolumab plus ipilimumab compared to chemotherapy. The most frequently reported grade 3 or higher serious treatment-related adverse events were colitis (3%), in the nivolumab plus ipilimumab arm, and anemia (2%) in the chemotherapy arm.

3.3 ICI-chemotherapy combination

The DREAM trial was a multicenter, single-arm, open-label, phase 2 trial conducted in 9 institutions in Australia [19]. In that study, 54 patients received cisplatin, pemetrexed, and durvalumab, in 3-week cycles, for up to 6 cycles. Durvalumab was continued for maintenance for up to 12 months. The primary endpoint was PFS at 6 months. Among 54 patients, 31 (57%; 95% CI: 44–70) were alive and progression-free at 6 months. The most frequent grade 3–4 adverse events were neutropenia (13%), nausea (11%), and anemia (7%). Five patients died during the study treatment, but none of the deaths were attributed to the study treatment.

The efficacy and safety of cisplatin, pemetrexed, and nivolumab were tested as first-line therapy for MPM in a phase II study, called JME-001 [20]. Cisplatin, pemetrexed, and nivolumab were administered intravenously every 3 weeks, for a total of 4 to 6 cycles. Patients that did not progress during the combination phase received maintenance therapy with nivolumab until disease progression or unacceptable toxicity. Among 18 enrolled patients, 14 (77·8%; 95% CI: 52·4–93·6) showed an objective response. Ten (55·6%) patients experienced grade 3 or worse adverse events, including disorders of metabolism or nutrition (33·3%), loss of appetite (27·8%), anemia (16·7%), and hyponatremia (11·1%). No treatment-related deaths occurred.

The efficacy and safety of pembrolizumab in combination with standard pemetrexed and platinum-based chemotherapy is currently being tested as a first-line treatment for MPM in phase II/III randomized study (NCT02784171) and in multicenter, open-label, non-randomized study (NCT04153565). Those results will be disclosed within a couple of years.

4. Future perspectives

Cisplatin plus pemetrexed has been the mainstay of systemic treatment for MPM. A phase III trial of platinum, pemetrexed plus the anti-VEGF inhibitor, bevacizumab, showed favorable results, with prolonged PFS and OS. The National Comprehensive Cancer Network (NCCN) guidelines advocate adding bevacizumab as an option;

Trial (Reference)	Phase	Primary endpoint	Drug	Number of patients	Histology	ORR (%) (CI)	median PFS (months) (CI)	median OS (months) (CI)
First-line								
MAPS [12]	III	OS	cisplatin + pemetrexed + bevacizumab	223	Epi: 179/223 (80%) non-Epi:44/223 (20%)	N.A.	9.2 (8.5–10.5)	18.8 (15.9–22.6)
			cisplatin + pemetrexed	225	Epi: 182/335 (81%) non-Epi:43/335(19%)	N.A.	7.3 (6.7–8.0)	16.1 (14.0–17.9)
Checkmate 743 [18]	III	OS	pembrolizumab	303	Epi: 229/303 (76%) non-Epi: 74/303 (24%)	40 (34.1–45.4)	6.8 (5.6–7.4)	18.1 (16.8–21.4)
			cisplatin + pemetrexed	302	Epi: 227/302 (75%) non-Epi: 75/302 (25%)	43 (37.1–48.5)	7.2 (6.9–8.0)	14.1 (12.4–16.2)
DREAM [19]	IIb	PFS	platinum + pemetrexed + durvalmab	54	Epi: 45/54 (83%) non-Epi: 9/54 (17%)	48 (35–6)	6.9 (5.5–9.0)	18.4 (13.1–24.8)
JME-001 [20]	II	ORR	cisplatin + pemetrexed + nivolumab	18	Epi: 14/18 (78%) non-Epi: 4/18 (22%)	78 (52.4–93.6)	8.0 (5.6–14.1)	20.8
Second-line or later								
MERIT [15]	IIb	ORR	nivolumab	34	Epi: 27 (79%) non-Epi: 7 (21%)	29 (17–46)	6.1 (2.9–9.9)	17.3 (11.5–N.R.)
MAPS2 [17]	III	If disease control was achieved in at least 40%	nivolumab + ipilimumab	62	Epi: 52 (83%) non-Epi: 11 (17%)	28 (16–40)	5.6 (3.1–8.3)	15.9 (10.7–N.R.)
			placebo	63	Epi: 53 (85%) non-Epi:9(15%)	19 (8–29)	4.0 (2.8–5.7)	11.9 (6.7–11.7)
RAMES [14]	II	OS	gemcitabine + ramcirumab	80	Epi: 68/80 (85%) non-Epi: 12 (15%)	6.3 (2–14)	6.4 (5.5–7.6)	13.8 (12.7–14.4)

Trial (Reference)	Phase	Primary endpoint	Drug	Number of patients	Histology	ORR (%) (CI)	median PFS (months) (CI)	median OS (months) (CI)
			gemcitabine	81	Epi: 70/81 (86%) non-Epi:11/81(14%)	10 (4–19)	7.5 (6.9–8.9)	7.5 (6.9–8.9)
CONFIRM [16]	III	PFS OS	nivolumab	221	Epi: 195/221 (88%) non-Epi: 26/221 (12%)	11 (N.A.)	3.0 (2.8–4.1)	10.2 (8.5–12.1)
			placebo	111	Epi: 98/111 (88%) non-Epi: 13/111 (12%)	1 (N.A.)	1.8 (1.4–2.6)	6.9 (5.0–8.0)

ORR: objective response rate; CI: confidence interval; PFS: progression-free survival; OS: overall survival; Epi: epithelioid; N.A.: not available; and DCR: disease control rate.

Table 1.
Recent clinical studies of systemic treatment in malignant pleural mesothelioma.

however, that regimen has not been approved in most countries. In recent years, ICIs have shown remarkable progress in treating MPM. Summaries of the major trials, with a focus on recent trials, are shown in **Table 1**. They include both salvage treatments and first-line treatments. Based on the CheckMate 743 trial results, the ICI-ICI combination of ipilimumab plus nivolumab could be considered a new standard front-line treatment.

Some unresolved problems should be investigated to make further improvements in the outcome of patients with MPM. One is the rapid drop-off in PFS observed among patients that receive ICIs. A recent study on patients with non-small cell lung cancer showed that ipilimumab plus nivolumab combined with 2 cycles of cytotoxic chemotherapy could reduce the rapid drop-offs in both PFS and OS [21]. Those results supported the notion that the ICI-chemotherapy combination should undergo further clinical development. Results are also anticipated from an ongoing trial that is testing a more aggressive strategy, with a combination of platinum, pemetrexed, atezolizumab, and bevacizumab (BEAT-meso, NCT03762018).

5. Conclusion

The results of various clinical trials that examined ICIs and angiogenesis inhibitors have been published in recent years. These trials have demonstrated better treatment options for MPM, but personalized medicine remains in the distant future. Although, MPM is a rare disease, the prognosis remains extremely poor. Therefore, it is necessary to conduct more clinical trials and translational investigations to establish personalized treatment options that can provide the most benefit to individual patients.

Acknowledgements

This study was supported by grants-in-aid from the Ministry of Health, Labor, and Welfare, Japan.

Conflict of interest

Dr. Fujimoto received consultancy fees from Boehringer Ingelheim, Ono, and Bristol-Myers Squibb, and honoraria or research funding from Chugai, Ono, Boehringer Ingelheim, Bristol-Myers Squibb, GlaxoSmithKline, and MSD.

Author details

Fumie Onishi and Nobukazu Fujimoto*
Department of Medical Oncology, Okayama Rosai Hospital, Okayama, Japan

*Address all correspondence to: nobufujimot@gmail.com

References

[1] Gemba K, Fujimoto N, Kato K, et al. National survey of malignant mesothelioma and asbestos exposure in Japan. Cancer Science. 2012;**103**:483-490. DOI: 10.1111/j.1349-7006.2011.02165.x

[2] Sharif S, Zahid I, Routledge T, et al. Extrapleural pneumonectomy or supportive care: Treatment of malignant pleural mesothelioma? Interactive Cardiovascular and Thoracic Surgery. 2011;**12**:1040-1045. DOI: 10.1510/icvts.2010.256289

[3] Zahid I, Sharif S, Routledge T, et al. Is pleurectomy and decortication superior to palliative care in the treatment of malignant pleural mesothelioma? Interactive Cardiovascular and Thoracic Surgery. 2011;**12**:812-817. DOI: 10.1510/icvts.2010.256271

[4] Kindler HL, Ismaila N, Armato SG 3rd, et al. Treatment of malignant pleural mesothelioma: American society of clinical oncology clinical practice guideline. Journal of Clinical Oncology. 2018;**36**:1343-1373. DOI: 10.1200/JCO.2017.76.6394

[5] Vogelzang NJ, Rusthoven JJ, Symanowski J, et al. Phase III study of pemetrexed in combination with cisplatin versus cisplatin alone in patients with malignant pleural mesothelioma. Journal of Clinical Oncology. 2003;**21**:2636-2644. DOI: 10.1200/JCO.2003.11.136

[6] Beebe-Dimmer JL, Fryzek JP, Yee CL, et al. Mesothelioma in the United States: A surveillance, epidemiology, and end results (SEER)-medicare investigation of treatment patterns and overall survival. Clinical Epidemiology. 2016;**8**:743-750. DOI: 10.2147/CLEP.S105396

[7] Langerak AW, De Laat PA, Van Der Linden-Van BCA, et al. Expression of platelet-derived growth factor (PDGF) and PDGF receptors in human malignant mesothelioma in vitro and in vivo. The Journal of Pathology. 1996;**178**:151-160. DOI: 10.1002/(SICI)1096-9896(199602)178:2<151::AID-PATH425>3.0.CO;2-E

[8] Honda M, Kanno T, Fujita Y, et al. Mesothelioma cell proliferation through autocrine activation of PDGF-betabeta receptor. Cellular Physiology and Biochemistry. 2012;**29**:667-674. DOI: 10.1159/000176386

[9] Till SJ, Francis JN, Nouri-Aria K, et al. Mechanisms of immunotherapy. The Journal of Allergy and Clinical Immunology. 2004;**113**:1025-1034. DOI: 10.1016/j.jaci.2004.03.024

[10] Finn OJ. Immuno-oncology: Understanding the function and dysfunction of the immune system in cancer. Annals of Oncology. 2012;**23**(Suppl 8):viii6-viii9. DOI: 10.1093/annonc/mds256

[11] Napoli F, Listi A, Zambelli V, et al. Pathological characterization of tumor immune microenvironment (TIME) in malignant pleural mesothelioma. Cancers (Basel). 2021;**13**:2564. DOI: 10.3390/cancers13112564

[12] Zalcman G, Mazieres J, Margery J, et al. Bevacizumab for newly diagnosed pleural mesothelioma in the mesothelioma Avastin Cisplatin Pemetrexed study (MAPS): A randomised, controlled, open-label, phase 3 trial. Lancet. 2016;**387**:1405-1414. DOI: 10.1016/S0140-6736(15)01238-6

[13] Scagliotti GV, Gaafar R, Nowak AK, et al. Nintedanib in

combination with pemetrexed and cisplatin for chemotherapy-naive patients with advanced malignant pleural mesothelioma (LUME-Meso): A double-blind, randomised, placebo-controlled phase 3 trial. The Lancet Respiratory Medicine. 2019;**7**:569-580. DOI: 10.1016/S2213-2600(19)30139-0

[14] Pinto C, Zucali PA, Pagano M, et al. Gemcitabine with or without ramucirumab as second-line treatment for malignant pleural mesothelioma (RAMES): A randomised, double-blind, placebo-controlled, phase 2 trial. The Lancet Oncology. 2021;**22**:1438-1447. DOI: 10.1016/S1470-2045(21)00404-6

[15] Okada M, Kijima T, Aoe K, et al. Clinical efficacy and safety of Nivolumab: Results of a multicenter, open-label, single-arm, Japanese phase II study in malignant pleural mesothelioma (MERIT). Clinical Cancer Research. 2019;**25**:5485-5492. DOI: 10.1158/1078-0432.CCR-19-0103

[16] Fennell DA, Ewings S, Ottensmeier C, et al. Nivolumab versus placebo in patients with relapsed malignant mesothelioma (CONFIRM): A multicentre, double-blind, randomised, phase 3 trial. The Lancet Oncology. 2021;**22**:1530-1540. DOI: 10.1016/S1470-2045(21)00471-X

[17] Scherpereel A, Mazieres J, Greillier L, et al. Nivolumab or nivolumab plus ipilimumab in patients with relapsed malignant pleural mesothelioma (IFCT-1501 MAPS2): A multicentre, open-label, randomised, non-comparative, phase 2 trial. The Lancet Oncology. 2019;**20**:239-253. DOI: 10.1016/S1470-2045(18)30765-4

[18] Baas P, Scherpereel A, Nowak AK, et al. First-line nivolumab plus ipilimumab in unresectable malignant pleural mesothelioma (CheckMate 743): A multicentre, randomised, open-label, phase 3 trial. Lancet. 2021;**397**:375-386. DOI: 10.1016/S0140-6736(20)32714-8

[19] Nowak AK, Lesterhuis WJ, Kok PS, et al. Durvalumab with first-line chemotherapy in previously untreated malignant pleural mesothelioma (DREAM): A multicentre, single-arm, phase 2 trial with a safety run-in. The Lancet Oncology. 2020;**21**:1213-1223. DOI: 10.1016/S1470-2045(20)30462-9

[20] Miyamoto Y, Kozuki T, Aoe K, et al. JME-001 phase II trial of first-line combination chemotherapy with cisplatin, pemetrexed, and nivolumab for unresectable malignant pleural mesothelioma. Journal for Immunotherapy of Cancer. 2021;**11**:e003288. DOI: 10.1136/jitc-2021-003288

[21] Paz-Ares L, Ciuleanu TE, Cobo M, et al. First-line nivolumab plus ipilimumab combined with two cycles of chemotherapy in patients with non-small-cell lung cancer (CheckMate 9LA): An international, randomised, open-label, phase 3 trial. The Lancet Oncology. 2021;**22**:198-211. DOI: 10.1016/S1470-2045(20)30641-0